MAGIC

in

HEALTH CARE

MAKING A DIFFERENCE
ONE MOMENT TO THE NEXT

Donna Devlin

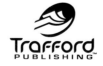

Trafford
PUBLISHING

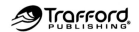

Praise for Donna Devlin

"I had the privilege of working with Donna during my time as Senior VP—Patient Experience. To say that I learned a great deal from her would be an understatement. This learning I have discovered subsequently came from not only watching Donna interact with some of the patients who had suffered bad outcomes (and the gentleness, the kindness and above all the humanizing aspect of that interaction) but also the fact that my own demons (Parkinson's disease) were far easier to bear—just by watching, and learning from this remarkable woman. Donna's *Magic Moments in Health Care* book will assist those of us in the healing professions to look at our behaviors with a new light; to approach these often difficult situations with a different paradigm. This small book can serve as a gentle reminder to do better. This is not a trivial thing this health care business—it is fraught with all sorts of trolls lying in wait for us and usually not under the bridge that we expect. We have professional colleges reminding us that we need to be competent, to not cross any boundaries; we have employers who on the surface seem not to comprehend what constitutes a safe number of staff—this text will assist everyone from the staff that hands out the supper trays to the head of cardiac. Thanks Donna for an inspiring yet practicable book on how to be your best in this grand endeavor called health care."

—Robert (Bob) V. Johnston MDCM, FRCPC *retired*
Emergency Physician, Director of Emergency Medicine,

Medical Director of Telehealth and Disaster Services, Chair of Medical Advisory Board, Chief Medical Officer and Senior VP, Member of Council of College of Physicians of Alberta, Senior VP of Patient Experience

"Donna Devlin's book, *Magic Moments in Health Care*, offers wise and heart-felt counsel that you will find deeply helpful whether you are just starting out in the health-care field or you've been working for decades. The stories of extraordinary empathy and bravery by the bedside of those who are suffering reveal the miracles that ordinary people can perform when moved by loving-kindness. Reading her book and contemplating the questions she raises will re-connect you with your original reasons for choosing a career helping those in physical and/or emotional need. Each of us as well as our loved ones will face illness in life; at those times may we all have care-givers--nurses, therapists, aides and doctors--who embody the approach taught so clearly in Donna's book."

—Lorne Ladner, Ph.D.,
author of *The Lost Art of Compassion*

"I have contracted Donna to deliver her "Magic Moments" workshops to careproviders in a variety of health care settings. Donna never fails to motivate and inspire her audiences with her messages that affirm the power and energy that each of us hold in making the journey of those we care for the best it can possibly be. There isn't a caregiver that won't appreciate these words of wisdom."

—Kim Frache,
Director Mental Health and Addictions Services,
Alberta Health Services

"With the numerous demands of staff, it is easy to become immobilized by the routines and tasks of our day, to a point where we forget how to truly engage with those we work with and those we care for. As leaders in health care, we need to remind ourselves that creating an environment of quality service, requires more that offering standardized approaches to care. We must also create a culture and environment that touches the spirit of individuals. I've embraced the philosophy of this book and encouraged staff to look for the simple ways they can create *magical moments*, every day. The impact has been powerful and has created a cultural shift in attitudes and behaviors. One's spirit truly does respond to kindness."

—Barbara J.P. Fredrich,
Quality and Service Development Manager and former
Continuing Care Centre Administrator, Carewest

"Your book is WONDERFUL!! Just as you exude so much energy and inspiration in all you do, this book captures the essence of the *"Magic"* that we all aspire to in healthcare and reminds us where to find it when it becomes lost ... as all magic tends to do when we forget to cherish it. It awakens the spirit within and reminds us of the reason we chose to enter the world of Healthcare in the first place...to create magic moments for those who need our help and in return gain magic moments that give us purpose and stay with us a lifetime. Thank-you for sharing these "magic moments" and giving insight and inspiration to renew the *"magic moments"* within me...within us all. I love it...what a wonderful message"

— Stephanie Keys RN. BScN,
Continuing Care Staff Educator, Carewest

Magic Moments-In Health Care

Making a difference one moment to the next

"Caretake this moment
Immerse yourself in its particulars
Respond to this person, this challenge, this deed. Quit the
evasions.
Stop giving yourself needless trouble
It is time to really live, to fully inhabit the situation you
happen to be in now." —*Epictetus*

Dedicated

To my dear husband Kent and my precious children Brenna, Calum, and Rhett who teach me about the beauty of magic everyday!

Acknowledgements

Stories are what guide us and inspire us in our life and work. We learn so much from each other. I am so very grateful to all the patients and healthcare workers that I have met who have shared their stories and time. It has been a privilege to serve those who were hurting and to walk amongst the most gracious people on earth—Health Care Workers. May you continue to be blessed in your journey of serving others. We need each other, and this became very apparent while I was writing this book.

I am forever grateful for my family's love, support, interest and encouragement. Mom, Dad, Kent, Brenna, Calum, Rhett and Jona, I always knew you were indeed my inspiration. To my friends and colleagues, Susan Parker, Kim Frache, Dr. Marlene Smart, Sue Melanson, Dr. Bob Johnston, Barbara Fredrich, Stephanie Keys, Colleen Doylend. I now know you cannot do great things without amazing people in your life to support, encourage and guide you all the way. With much love and gratitude to you all, and may we all bask in the magic around us!

Contents

A Note from the Author

For the purpose of this book I will use the words: "patients" and "residents" interchangeably. These terms could apply to any person you provide care for.

I also use the terms: helpers, caregivers, healthcare professionals, healthcare workers, healthcare staff interchangeably. These terms could apply to anyone providing care.

Some of the stories in the book have been altered and names changed to protect the identities and enhance the message.

The pine cone on the front cover symbolizes, *"The huge potential in small things."* It is also a medical symbol that dates back to the early 14th century. The heart symbol in early medical illustrations was first shaped like pine cones in the Hippocratic School by Galen.

"Magic is about transforming our self and work in health care from one moment to the next."

—*Donna Devlin*

Preface

THE NEED OF MAGIC MOMENTS

"The practice of medicine is an art, not a trade; a calling, not a business; a calling in which your heart will be exercised equally with your head."

—Sir William Osler

I have worked twenty-five years as a healthcare professional. For the past twelve years, I have had the privilege of working with healthcare staff in an educational, staff development capacity. Like you, I am on a journey of finding and creating meaning in my life and work. No two journeys are alike, but there are common threads that bind healthcare professionals together. Those of us in the helping profession are continually faced with increasing pressure, strain, and a more hectic pace. The hurdles we must constantly overcome sometimes cause us to feel frustrated, exhausted and inadequate. There are times when we become depleted and disillusioned with our work. This book identifies our challenges and acknowledges the difficulties we face on a daily basis. The stories I share are ones to which most healthcare professionals can relate. Our patients need to feel human contact and connection. This is not always an easy thing to achieve. We sometimes become so focused on our tasks, technology and routines that our jobs become mechanical and meaningless. It seems to me that what is fundamentally lacking is honoring the sacredness of our mere presence. We need to truly honor those moments when we know we are connecting with someone or have done everything we possibly can to make a connection. There may be times, because of the nature of a patient's illness, when we feel like we're not making a meaningful connection because our experience isn't as positive and warm as we think it should be. But I believe in all these cases, we do make a connection—one of understanding and compassion. This is especially important with our so-called "difficult" or "challenging" patients and families.

This process of honoring the magic moments must begin with defining the term "magic" and understanding our role as healthcare workers. I believe each of us yearn for that connection where we know we are making a difference in the life of another human being. I also believe that there are certain hurdles in healthcare that can hinder our helping journey. Acknowledging and identifying hurdles like "the helper's hole," the difficult patient, our fears, worries, doubts and egos will set the stage toward honoring the mode of magic moments on our healthcare journey. I refer to these as "Magic Moment Modes," which are natural, conscious, transformative, replenishing processes involving perspective and knowledge. The modes of magic moments involve bringing conscious awareness into our work and creating an environment that honors the significance of serving others. Ultimately, this is where we derive our meaning as health care professionals.

The stories shared in this book illustrate the tools we have to create magic in our work and encourage all of us to remember why we have chosen to do this work. The exercises and questions will gently guide us to further explore our roles as healthcare workers. The concepts in this book may not be new, yet my hope is that they will inspire and rejuvenate you, whether you are in the beginning, middle or end of your journey as a healthcare professional.

As healthcare professionals, we walk a line involving sorrow, joy, frustration and amazement. Every day we find ourselves in the humbling position of making a difference in the lives of others. And that is no small accomplishment. This book was written for all those healthcare professionals who walk this line every day in the service of others in need. It was written to acknowledge, inspire and encourage healthcare professionals on their journey of serving others.

You may have been drawn to or encouraged to read this book. If it causes you to reflect upon yourself or your work, or provides you with a strategy going forward, or encourages you, inspires you or renews your faith in what it means to be a healthcare worker, my mission has been accomplished. If you encourage others to read it or you reread it yourself, then I have been successful beyond my wildest dreams. Many blessings to you, and may you continue to grow in your work. Know that you alone can make a difference in the lives of others. And that is no small wonder...it is magic!

1

MAGIC MOMENTS

"There are two ways to live your life—one is as though nothing is a miracle, the other is as though everything is a miracle."

—ALBERT EINSTEIN

Rodger's Dictionary defines magic as *"art, producing effects-by assisting or master of secret force; having the power of effect."* A moment is defined by Rodgers dictionary as *"a minute portion of time, an instant, importance, influence of effect."*

It is *quality* of time, not quantity, which enables health care workers to acknowledge that we alone have the potential to create meaning in our work and transform our workplace. It is not uncommon for people to go through life and work as if they are on autopilot, neither truly valuing nor experiencing the sacredness of what it means to be alive and fully engaged in living. We exist but have difficulty understanding the meaning of creating magic and honoring each moment.

When we think of magic, we usually think of something esoteric, out of this world, out of our grasp or reach. However, there is magic in the everyday and the ordinary. We all have a secret force that can create magic. This secret force is part of our consciousness and compassion. We need to remember and honor all our moments of connection. There is value in these moments, however ephemeral they may seem.

A magic moment is not about caring for the moment and more about caring in the moment. It is about *being present* in those moments. We may say, "Of course I am present. I am in the room providing their care, am I not?" But are we really present, or are we there in body only? Do we hear the patient speaking to us but unable to truly grasp or concentrate on what they are saying? Are we thinking about how we are going to answer or who we have to see in the next room? We may smile and nod our heads, but can our patients detect our preoccupation and vacancy in our eyes? We may not realize we are doing this, but we have all had moments like this in our work. We have either been on the receiving end of that preoccupied look, or we may have unknowingly provided that look to those in our care.

For the purposes of this book, magic involves creating and honoring moments at work with a conscious, compassionate open approach. We are co-creating the type of work environment we want that is not influenced by external demands. We have to go within ourselves and search for ways to honor and create magic moments while caring for others. Magic also involves appreciating the good stuff that occurs so we can continue to create more of it!

Interestingly enough, we are more apt to share moments of frustration and discouragement with other staff than "good stuff" or magic moments. We don't often hear staff members saying, "I had the most incredible moment with a patient! There was this connection. I knew that I was making a difference. I may not have been curing their illness, but my presence there was easing and comforting and even healing." More often, we may hear statements like "I am looking after the most miserable, cantankerous, frustrating person who won't cooperate. I am too busy and underpaid for this."

Magic Moments are about what we focus our attention on in healthcare. Are we focusing on what we can do or on what we can't do? In this book we will look at valuing the sacredness in patient interactions and exploring modes to develop and honor more of those moments as a means of getting in touch with the real essence of our work; the human essence, the spirit.

The very first step in creating magic moments is to understand ourselves. Understanding ourselves will help us realize when we are in "the hole" (more about this in Chapter Four) and help us stay out of the hole. This is very difficult in itself. It may be easy to see when other colleagues and staff are in the hole yet it is very difficult to recognize this in ourselves. Patterns of thinking and behaving can become so entrenched in how we cope that we need to scrub them off once in awhile to see clearly.

Our best tool for creating magic moments is ourselves. We can create amazing work moments when we focus on what we have instead of what we don't have. Therefore, it is essential for us to examine who we are as healthcare workers before we start this process of creating and honoring the magic moments in our work.

Questions to Ponder

- What is the good stuff in helping?
- How often do you share the good stuff?

- What are you paying attention to?
- What are you accentuating?
- What do you focus your time and energy on during the day?

It's easy to become so focused on the "difficulties" that we miss opportunities to create magic and we then will allow our whole day to become miserable, instead of just acknowledging the difficult encounter and creating magic amongst the difficulty.

Cindy, an emergency room nurse related a story of a very demanding patient in the waiting room. She explained that most of the staff ignored him because they believed he did not understand that they were busy and had more urgent patients to attend to. The staff made no eye contact and avoided acknowledging his concerns. This patient became increasingly agitated and very belligerent. It became obvious that the situation was starting to escalate and that there was a potential for violence. A staff member, named Roberta wasn't directly involved in the escalation, and decided to approach the patient with a glass of water and to sit down with him. The patient started to relax and then broke down crying. The patient said to Roberta, "I just wanted someone to see me, you know, to look at me, and not just say we are busy with more urgent patients." He went on to add, "I know they are busy, but I felt I was just a nuisance to them and that I didn't matter."

The Department now has a philosophy where being a patient starts when a person walks in the door. Staff are to say something as simple as, "Hello" and share a genuine, "I see you smile." Staff also provides additional usually somewhat repetitive information as to when the patient might be seen. Staff started to note a decrease in frustrated and angry patients in the waiting room with this type of approach. The angry and difficult patients were not totally eliminated, for this is the very nature of our work to assist those in need of care without judgment and that doesn't just mean the pleasant people.

Questions to Ponder

- Are we too busy for the hellos?
- Are we so overwhelmed that we don't take the time to acknowledge and then inadvertently create more tension in the workplace?
- How many times have we been on the receiving end of service from someone that didn't even lift their head up to look at us? What was that like?
- How many times did you meet a health care professional and they didn't even introduce themselves? What was that like? Why was it important to know their name?

Allison is an adult student, wife and mother studying to become a nurse. Having no idea what I do for a living or what book I was writing, she shared some observations with me one day.

"You know, Donna, I have been told from the more "seasoned" staff that all this compassion I have for others in need isn't going to last forever."

When I asked Alison what she thought of this, she responded, "Compassionate, kind and big-hearted is who I am. How do you lose compassion along the way?"

"What do you do for yourself so you can keep giving to others so unselfishly?" I asked.

"Oh, I take time for myself, through baths, solitude and I seek out support when I need it, and more than that, I look for moments during my shift where I am not just giving I am receiving. There is nothing more fulfilling than when you are holding someone's hands and you look them in the eyes and they say, 'Someone must have wished you to me.' I think the seasoned ones miss the refilling by avoiding eye contact and not taking a moment to really see the person." Alison went on to add that she believes "There are people who give care to others and reap the benefits of giving. Not a shift goes by without a beautiful happening. How open are our hearts when we enter our workplace? Should we not be looking at it as a gift we have been given, to serve others, to show love, mercy and companionship to another in their most crucial time in life? Do unto others as you would have them do unto you!"

Alison's comments are so profound that they still echo through me. It is interesting to note her choice of the word "enter." Are we "entering" with our presence, or are we on the way out before we even get there?

Do unto others as you would have them do unto you. Such a simple statement that we have all heard many times before. Yet, like so many things in life, we sometimes miss the true message or trivialize it as jargon. Repeat this message, and this time let it resonate within you. What does it mean when you say it again? What images are conjured up as you think of moments when you provided care?

2

WHO ARE YOU?

"Self awareness is the most important thing you bring into your work."

—Sandra Butler

Who we are is a vital component of our work as a healthcare professional. Self-awareness helps us understand how we cope and respond to situations in the helping field. Being aware of our thoughts, feelings and behaviors and how they influence our interactions will enable us to become more compassionate caregivers. Who we are as healthcare workers will greatly influence our ability to create and honor magic moments at work.

There will be times and situations in our personal and work life that will cause us to feel depleted, meaningless and worthless, so before we can understand our patients and make a difference in the moment, we must understand and be able to help ourselves. To do this, we must be able to identify and acknowledge what makes us vulnerable, as well as our strengths and ways to refuel, restore, and reframe. If we want to make a change, self awareness can give us the self-confidence and self-esteem to engage in this process. Self awareness brings us closer in line with our values and purposes as healthcare workers. Becoming self-aware is a lifelong process that needs constant attention. A crucial part of this is not accepting unhappy situations and being willing to search out alternatives for perceiving and coping with difficult situations.

Self-awareness gives us options for growth, influences our success and increases our ability to respond authentically to others. Self-awareness has been described as our "emotional intelligence," something that studies are proving invaluable to our personal and professional success in the workplace. Daniel Goldman, author of *Working with Emotional Intelligence*, identifies emotional intelligence as "enabling the worker in developing greater skills in areas such as initiative, motivation, self regulation, empathy, and service orientation." These skills are crucial in our quest to finding meaning in every moment.

A.W. Combs and colleagues at the University of Florida conducted research on the characteristics of effective helpers and concluded: "Good helpers are not born, nor are they made in the sense of being taught. Becoming a helper is a time-consuming process. It is not simply a matter of learning methods or acquiring gadgets and gimmicks. It is a deeply personal process of exploration and discovery, the growth of unique individuals learning over a period of time how to use themselves effectively for helping other people."

Caregivers don't often take the opportunity to ask themselves questions that would help them on the road to finding meaning and magic moments in their work. Our search as caregivers is an inward exploration of self for an outward service to others. Every encounter with another person in need is a reflection of our deepest values and thoughts. Conflict arises in us when our action towards others is in direct contrast to what we value and hold dear. There is enormous value in asking ourselves exploratory questions.

Who we are as helpers becomes amplified through the relationships we create with our patients. We can discover a lot about ourselves through our helping relationships.

A *Course in Miracles* clearly reflects this with the following:

> "When you meet anyone, remember it is a holy encounter. As you see him, you will see yourself, as you treat him, you will treat yourself. As you think of him, you will think of yourself. Never forget this, for in him you will either find yourself or lose yourself."
>
> —*Schueman and Thetford*

Self-Awareness Exercise

✓ What motivated you to become a healthcare worker?
✓ What brought you into this kind of work?
✓ What are your goals, hopes, and expectations? What is your mission?
✓ What are your emotional buttons? These are your sensitivities and vulnerabilities and troublesome helping moments.
✓ Think about a helping situation past/ present. What is your degree of involvement? Has it changed as you worked in the field?
✓ What are your Awesome Helping moments? (This answers why you do this difficult work) Ah, this is why I'm doing this!! Take time to write down your most fulfilling moment as a healthcare worker.

✓ What are your strengths and stretches or challenges as a health care professional?

✓ How does your personality influence your interaction?

Understanding additional aspects of "therapeutic use of self" is an important asset in the creation of magic moments. The questions in this next exercise are based in part on the principles of Dr. Carl Rogers' work involving humanistic person-centered approaches to therapeutic relationship. I would define "therapeutic" as not necessarily curing but more of a healing and easing that comforts and encourages emotional, physical, mental and spiritual health and the highest level of functioning for our patients. For some of you, this may be your first encounter with these principles; for others this will serve as a good reminder.

Therapeutic Self-Assessment

✓ Can I be perceived as trustworthy?

✓ Can I communicate clearly with out ambiguity?

✓ Can I have a positive respectful attitude towards this person that has compassion, acceptance and warmth? Or do I only accept the some aspects of their behaviors and feelings and disapprove of the others?

✓ Can I be aware of the need to be separate yet enter the patient world and see it with understanding and empathy? Or am I afraid of this closeness with another human being and become indifferent cold and rejecting?

✓ Is my need to be liked so great that I become offended and upset by hostile rude and uncooperative patients?

✓ Do I feel inferior and cover with an act of superiority?

✓ To feel important and worthy do I keep the patient dependent on me?

For most of us in the field of healthcare, helping is a natural way of being. We have a desire and a need to be of help to someone. If we can get out of our own way, get past our thoughts, judgments and assumptions, and do what we do best—helping someone in their time of need—who we are becomes clearer to us. Understanding ourselves puts us in the best position to be consciously present and able to respond to the needs of our patients. One unknown author says, "Sometimes the best way to figure out who you are is to get to that place where you don't have to be anything else."

HURDLES IN HELPING

3

OLD BAGGAGE

"The truth is that our finest moments are most likely to occur when we are feeling deeply uncomfortable, unhappy, or unfulfilled. For it is only in such moments, propelled by our discomfort, that we are likely to step out of our ruts and start searching for different ways or truer answers."

—M. Scott Peck

Now that we have had the chance to understand ourselves better, let's look at the barriers and extra "baggage" that we carry. Thinking back to the nursing student's comment on "seasoned staff," I can't help but wonder if we are "ripe and rotten, or green and growing."

Healthcare workers face serious challenges every day. We are understaffed with limited resources and our workload is always being increased. Health management systems are constantly undergoing enormous change and reorganization. Quality in the workplace and support of each other seems to be lacking. We are suffering and have to cope with the fallout. The baggage is amplified as a result of all these challenges and the disillusionment with the hectic, chaotic field of healthcare.

Our biggest resource is ourselves, so we need to consider what we can do to help ourselves and those we care for. This will take commitment, perseverance and a willingness to not accept the current status quo and create and honor the essence of our work. This will involve, reframing and focusing on what *can* be done instead of what can't be done. We must look at ways we can cope and thrive through the chaos. Our ability to look at what is in our control and how we can positively influence each day, moment to moment, is paramount.

Some might believe this is a Pollyanna approach and avoids the "real issue." However, the "real" issue is being present for those in our care with compassion and kindness! The Magic lies in that we do have what it takes to move through our fears to a greater connection with ourselves and those we serve. Our fears can prevent us from giving this gift of ourselves, our presence. We can and do create this amongst the confusion. We do amazing work, and with practice and determination we will continue to focus on what really matters in healthcare and not get caught up into in the chaos and be limited by our disabling "baggage."

The following list identifies a list of baggage that prevents healthcare providers from making a meaningful connection with someone in their care and not growing in their work. See if you can relate to any of these thoughts and ideas. Is there some baggage you would add to the list? Do you detect a common theme? What is it? *What baggage would you have to get rid of in order to make a magic moment connection with your patient?*

- Fear that you will make the patient feel worse
- Fear that you don't have the right skills
- Fear that you are lacking

- Fear that you will make a mistake
- Fear that you may get hurt either physically or mentally
- Fear of being overly attached
- Fear of what others think of you
- Fear of appearing foolish
- Belief that nothing I can say or do will change this residents/patients reality
- I am in a hurry
- Not enough time
- Not enough help
- Lack of confidence
- Self conscious
- Physical fatigue
- Always listening to others complaining- holding me back
- Intellectual snobbery- assuming that other people know
- Overwhelmed
- Gossip
- Hardness
- Reluctance to let people at work know them very well for fear of inadequacy
- Impatience
- Stereotyping
- Personal issues on mind
- External and internal demands

This list clearly identifies that we are somehow lacking, that we aren't enough or we don't have enough. We may wonder if what we are doing will truly make a difference. Can you see the common themes of inadequacy, self-doubt, fear and helplessness? Helpers don't like to feel helpless. Acknowledging and letting go of our extra carry-on luggage allows us to connect with our patients and create Magic moments!

Freeing Fear

It is hard to imagine or admit that, yes, we caregivers are sometimes afraid. We are supposed to be the fearless that go boldly where others fear to tread. That is why so many "outsiders" ask caregivers questions like "How and why do you do this work that you do?" How do you deal with human suffering, pain and death?" "Don't you find your work depressing?" These questions support the "super helping myth" that nothing bothers us and that we can do all and be all to those in our care. Fear can take on many shapes for helpers, but generally speaking, themes of fears emerge as: "They" (our patients, managers, and colleagues) will find out that I am not as good as I appear to be." This is the "imposter syndrome," something females in particular tend to experience, or at least they are more apt to acknowledge this experience.

Healthcare workers have a tremendous fear of making an error. We worry and fear that we may have done or said the wrong thing. Dale G. Larson's book, *The Helper's Journey*, describes the "terror of error," something we healthcare workers all understand. It is 3:00 AM and we should be in a deep sleep, yet we are fraught with worry and fear we have made a drug error, procedural error or wrong diagnosis. We wake up at night wondering if we gave the correct dose or locked the narcotic cupboard. In workshops I refer to this as the "misery of mistakes."

The word "misery" comes from the Latin word *miseria*, or miser, which means wretchedness. The word "miser" has to do with hoarding and "hanging on to things." Often it is the most sensitive and reflective staff that experience the greatest misery after a mistake. We have all made mistakes in our work as healthcare professionals. We are only human, except that when we make a mistake it can be life-threatening or life-altering. The misery occurs when we blame ourselves or hold on to or hide our mistakes. The truth is, we can learn from our mistakes and also learn to let go of them. When we make a mistake, it's important to acknowledge the emotional impact of it, talk about it with our colleagues and forgive ourselves.

As caregivers, we make thousands of decisions and judgment calls every day. As much as we would like to believe there are absolutes in our work, in reality there are hundreds of shades of gray in the middle. We must rely upon our training and skills to make decisions in the best interests of those in our care. In one of my favorite movies, *National Velvet*, there are messages for us in the most surprising places. At one point, the trainer says to his young groom, "You can make a wrong decision for the right reason or a right decision for the wrong reason—who is to say which is right?" This certainly applies to most caregivers.

We also feel pressure from advances in technology. New technological demands increase our fears dramatically. Nothing is changing more rapidly in healthcare than technology. We no sooner learn one procedure and treatment before it becomes obsolete. We don't have enough time to fully understand how to properly utilize the equipment before being proficient in it.

Sometimes we also fear for our own wellbeing. There is a certain amount of physical risk involved as a healthcare worker, for example, being contaminated by AIDS, hepatitis or SARS, or being assaulted by a violent patient. In many cases, however, we are also assaulted emotionally—being the recipients of harsh, condemning words from those we care for. We can grieve, suffer and feel emotionally drained and consumed by those in our care. This is when we really need the support of our colleagues and management.

Early in my nursing career I worked in an intensive psychiatric care unit. I will never forget the day I was assigned to a woman in room 46B. I had heard that she was in delirium tremors due to alcohol abuse. She was physically and verbally aggressive. Nothing could have prepared me for my encounter with her or the fear I felt when I entered her room. I peaked into her room and there she was, a very large woman with all four limbs restrained. She raised her head a little, looked at me and said, "Hi, sweetie" in the kindest, calmest voice. She added, "Would you be kind enough to untie just one hand so I can scratch a spot on my back?" She looked miserable and calm so I thought untying one restraint would be safe enough. I proceeded to untie her left hand restraint, and before I could respond she grabbed me by my collar and in a threatening voice said, "Now I am going to beat the sh— out of you." It is quite amazing, since it all happened so quickly. I managed to swallow my fear and using a lighthearted, humorous approach, I said, "Ah, Mrs. Starch, I am wearing white and what a bloody mess that would be." She immediately released my collar and throat and said, "Why, yes. We can't have that, can we?" I immediately replaced the restraint.

Often when healthcare workers feel fear and anxiety, it is because they believe they have been thrown into a situation for which they are ill-prepared. We may feel "stretched too thin" and overwhelmed by the severity and sheer volume of the tasks at hand. Training, education and support will help to alleviate some of this fear.

Fear grows and thrives in the cold dark places that see no light. Bringing light to our fears will diminish its power over us. If we are afraid to tell someone about our fears and pretend that nothing really bothers us, our fears will grow and fester and manifest in other parts of our life. We need to truly believe that we can feel the fear and do what we need to do anyway. This in itself becomes very freeing. Remember, our fears are only as debilitating as we allow them to be. When I feel fear I recognize it as a marker that tells me, "Hey, this is something I have to do to move forward."

Healthcare workers must make a conscious decision to deal with fear. In order to do this, we need to acknowledge and express our fear then gain knowledge and take positive action. If we don't properly manage fear or let it go, fear will explode in us and manifest in all sorts of gremlin ways. Busting fear and building courage are choices. *Free* your fear! Let it go.

F – First off, acknowledge your fear and what you are afraid of.

R – Replace your fear response with one of courage and action instead of reaction. Replace your fearful thoughts with those of power. You say 50,000 things to yourself each day. What are you telling yourself? Find out more information and gain knowledge and skills. Writing down your fears is a powerful step towards managing them.

E – Engage in an activity that helps to ground and comfort you. Talk it out with supportive colleagues. Breathing becomes a marker to get in touch with the present. Since your fears usually have to do with the past or future, we can use our breath awareness to live in the moment and move forward valiantly.

E – Expect the best. Have a relationship with a higher source that guides and helps you.

Questions to Ponder

- How does your fear manifest in you? What are your usual responses? Do you avoid or respond physically, etc.?
- What do you need to learn more about to feel more comfortable and less fearful?
- How do you ground yourself to the present when you are stressed?
- What techniques do you need to learn to deal with fears, real and imagined?
- How can your mission and values guide you during your shift?

4

THE HELPER'S HOLE

"We cannot live only for ourselves. A thousand fibers connect us with our fellow men; and along these fibers, as sympathetic threads, our actions run as cause, and they come back as effects."

—HERMAN MELVILLE

There is a fear that if we do give the gift of ourselves, we will fall into the "helper's hole" and never get out. So the challenge becomes how do we give the gift of ourselves and still maintain separateness so we don't fall in the hole? Falling in the helper's hole is the easy part. Staying out and knowing when we are about to fall in is the difficult part.

"The hole" is a metaphor for our helping relationships. A hole is defined as a "cavity, gap, break or something hollow." Magic moments happen when we make a caring connection with those in our care. The "helping hole" refers to the inability to make this connection and where we, as well as the patients, are left feeling hollow or with feelings of lack and want. The hole can also be when our patients are suffering or in pain. At times we may not notice the hole yet experience symptoms of falling into it: we feel hurt, consumed, underappreciated, tired or useless and believe we are incapable of providing "good care." (It is interesting to note that it seems easier to recognize when our colleagues are in the hole than when we are.) At other times, we notice the hole and for some unknown reason we fall headlong into it with our patient.

There will be times in our helping career where our sense of being able to help is in peril. We walk a fine line when we make this connection with those we are helping. We know it is the patient's journey, not ours. Our role becomes one of serving others and not taking on their pain or suffering. We know when we have made a Magic connection with our patient; there is a blurring between us and the patient. This connection is indescribable. It's as if time stands still and a barrier has been knocked down. There is a sense of complete knowing, compassion and understanding that we are all the same. It is a feeling of being filled up, a kind of "goose bump" experience.

A mere thread connects us to these feelings of compassion and understanding that go beyond words. This thread is invisible, vulnerable and universal. It is a need to help another human being in distress. It is not just performing the procedures and treatment (which, of course, are very important); it is the pure essence of being with someone in their darkest moments and that person knowing we are there for them. In this way, we use ourselves as a tool to comfort and heal.

We caregivers constantly walk a tightrope of caring, balancing what others need from us and what we need for ourselves. When we over-identify with those in our care and no longer have a life separate from those in our care, we become predisposed to falling in the hole. On the other hand, some of us feel like blocks of ice, unaffected by our exposure to someone in need. Our challenge will always be to find the compassionate empathetic place in the middle where we find meaning as helpers.

Symptoms of Falling into the Helper's Hole

We have all experienced these symptoms at some point in our helping career. The key to understanding these symptoms is to determine the extent and length of time that we have been experiencing these symptoms.

- Irritability/anger with those around us
- Blame- patients, family, system and co-workers
- Feelings of being overwhelmed and consumed
- Difficulty in sleeping and preoccupation with thoughts of work
- Cynicism/negativity and detachment from those in your care
- Cold, flu, stomachache, headache and backache that won't go away
- Difficulty concentrating and remembering
- Sadness, weepiness and depressive thoughts and feelings
- Continual fatigue
- Less satisfied with helping efforts
- Perfectionism- believing we are the only one who can help those in distress
- Guilt /fear
- Helplessness
- Not eating a healthy diet for lack of time
- Not exercising and taking care of physical health
- Over use of alcohol or increase in smoking

- Losing connection with family and friends and taking no time to socialize

Early in my nursing career, I was counseling a woman whose toddler had just died from a genetic condition. Her infant had just been diagnosed with the same condition, and she had just found out that her husband had been having an affair throughout their entire marriage. Looking back now, I can see that I was unable to help this woman after a certain point because I had begun to over-identify with her suffering and had fallen into the hole with her. I found myself feeling bitter toward the husband and overly sad for her. At the time, I remember thinking that she was my age and that this could happen to me. She reminded me of myself.

The people we are trying to help do not want us in the hole with them! If they could, they would probably shout at us, "Get out of this hole! This is my hole!"

Caregivers in the hole with their patients only make their patients feel more vulnerable and hopeless. Our patients don't want us in the hole with them! For our own wellbeing, as well as theirs, it is best to be with them yet not take on their pain and situation. We can only do this if we feel in balance ourselves. When we feel exhausted and depleted, there is a higher risk of falling into the hole. Naturally, we try to avoid this. Unfortunately, in these cases, we end up having no connection with the patient. I'm sure we can all relate to these feelings of exhaustion, preoccupation and confusion, all of which make us feel that we are on a one-way street going the wrong way and are about to be hit. Most helpers just keep going and are uncomfortable asking for help or assistance.

It is much easier for caregivers to give help than to receive it. Someone at a workshop once said to me, "If you say yes to everything, what is your yes worth?" Keep in mind that No is just a two-letter word. Sometimes when we are asked to do the extra shift or volunteer to bake cookies for our child's school fundraiser, it's okay to say no! In fact, saying no can be essential for our well-being. It is in our best interests to say No often. That way, when we do say yes, it will be with resounding enthusiasm.

One of the biggest problems with No is that it causes us to feel enormous guilt. Yes, guilt—the gift that keeps on giving. It is only after years of practicing—yes, practicing!—that I can now say it. Practicing involves consciously using the word in different situations and observing the results in yourself and your life. I might still experience some guilt for a few minutes, but nothing compared to saying yes to something and then worrying and fretting about how I would accomplish it in the timeframe allotted. My aim is to have no guilt, and I am well on the way to being guilt-liberated!

5

EGO, LABELS AND JUDGEMENT

"We look for solutions in many places,
but where is the solution?
The solution is in the human heart."

—AUTHOR UNKNOWN

Ego

We want to make a difference in our work, so what would prevent us from doing so? Our number-one stumbling block is ourselves and the thoughts associated with ourselves—our ego. Author Eckart Tolle says that "Whenever you feel superior or inferior to anyone, that's the ego in you." He also says, "You can value and care for things, but whenever you get attached to things, you will know it is the ego."

What exactly is the ego? The term is used frequently, yet what does it mean? Our ego is that voice inside our head that constantly focuses on either the past or the future, never the present. Our ego traps us with thoughts like "There isn't enough time or staff to make a difference;" "I don't know what to do anyway, and no matter what, it won't be enough." The ego is not wrong or bad (that would be the ego talking!); it just is. Knowing that our ego is a part of us and how it can manifest in our life and limit us from who we really are, gives us the power to tame it. When we know that we are truly more than we think we are and that we have more than enough to make a difference in the life of another, we have tamed our ego.

We are so much more than our ego! In fact, we are not our ego at all. The ego is full of wanting and needing and leads us to believe that everything is about us. One of the key markers to falling in the hole is thinking that a resident's situation is about us. It not about us; it is about them. Even when we wish residents could do things themselves because we're so busy, it's not about us. It is about them and their needs. Can we truly accept the state patients are in without judgment? (Of course, none of this will matter, and we will not get this concept, if we are feeling depleted.)

We are often our own worst critics. We know the voice of our ego very well and that voice knows us very well. During times of vulnerability and strain, when the ego calls our name, we invariably answer, "Yes, you are right. I am not enough, and there isn't enough…" This is a self-depleting cycle. Even if we manage to pull ourselves out of this cycle and start the process of believing that we are enough and that we have enough, someone on our team will be quick to point out, "Hey, remember, we don't have enough, and you aren't enough; the patients are more than enough, so don't be thinking that this moment is enough…" This is all the more reason to surround ourselves with people who acknowledge that "enough is enough;" or who think "I am enough;" "I have enough;" "This moment is enough." With a kind voice, we can acknowledge to ourselves that enough is enough, that we have done all we can with kindness and compassion. Unfortunately, because we feel so overwhelmed, we think we've fallen short and failed to provide our patients with all the compassion and kindness they need.

Author Ken Blanchard said, "The biggest problem in business today is the human ego, which pushes God out and puts you in the center." Spirituality acknowledges that there is something more important than we are, something more loving than we are, a higher power than ourselves that can give people peace.

The ego is a big factor that impedes our ability to connect with ourselves and others. Much of what prevents healthcare workers from making a connection with those in their care originates from the ego, which effectively controls how we think about ourselves and others and is filled with judgments and labels.

Judgments and Labels

Do we judge patients before we see them and then continue judging them at every encounter? Are we aware of how and when we judge patients?

Since so much of our work is tied up with identifying problems and seeking solutions, the search for the true essence of our patients may fall by the wayside. Instead, we focus on their problems, or what we believe their problems to be. We forget that their heart condition or brain disease is not who they really are. Sometimes we must look really deep to see their true essence. What drives them? What comforts them? What are their hopes and fears and dreams? It is hard to imagine that someone with a debilitating illness or even a palliative situation can have dreams, yet they can and do. We tend to make assumptions about their situation. According to Professor David Peters, "The microscope is good at seeing genes, but the person is disappearing from the doctor's view."

Labels are commonly used in healthcare. These descriptions or expectations usually involve some judgment of an object, event or person, which feeds our need to be right, superior, etc. At some point, we all may have used the following to describe patients: senile, pain-in-the-neck, sweetie pie, paranoid, neurotic, manipulative, know-it-all, whiner, miserable, cantankerous. We judge ourselves and others. The voice inside our head is often the sniper and critic. "I am stupid...incompetent... lame...dumpy...ridiculous..." Our judgments and labels become self- fulfilling prophesies. All of a sudden, the label that we use to describe a patient becomes our reality. The "manipulative person" becomes manipulative, and so on.

Sara, a patient on a medical unit, had the staff frustrated, annoyed and angry. Some staff believed she was demanding and "ornery." Any request Sara had for help was seen in this light. It is interesting to note that the more the staff labeled and judged Sara as ornery, the more difficult or ornery she seemed to become. The staff who described her as "afraid and anxious" saw her with more compassion and in a different light. As a result, their experience with her was different from that of the staff who labeled her as ornery.

It can be normal practice on some units to label patients. To fit in, we may inadvertently accentuate these traits, which can cause more difficulty during a shift. To avoid this, we must learn to catch ourselves and observe our language, thoughts and descriptive words. Spend one entire shift with awareness of the words we use and keep track of the thoughts that cross our mind.

In healthcare, we often label patients by their diagnoses instead of their names and then fail to notice that this is all we see in them. Our challenge is to look into their eyes, especially those of difficult patients, and see their essence, the human spirit beyond their diagnoses and illnesses. I have found that when I am particularly afraid or frustrated with a patient and force myself to really look the person in the eye, I see something that I scramble to find words for—their essence, their humanness. Maybe the reason we avoid eye contact with them is that we are afraid to see the essence of another human being. I don't believe for one minute that we could treat another harshly or without compassion if we saw ourself in that person's eyes. We would see our reflection and know that we are all one.

We seem to have unintentionally separated from people in our care by labeling them. That is how we make sense out of some the patient situations in which we find ourselves. As a result, Mr. Edwards is no longer Mr. Edwards; he is the irritating, congested heart failure patient in room 24B. Mable is no longer Mable but the anxious, demanding woman in the room across from the nursing station. We have all used these terms to some extent. It has become such a normal way of operating that we may not even know we're doing it. We believe these labels somehow help us to cope with difficult people, however, in the end they only cause us to feel more drained, negative, cynical and inadvertently detached from those we are trying to help. When we consciously or unconsciously use labels in care, we inadvertently add to an already tense situation. Patients believe we don't care about them, and they are partly right—because of our fear, ego, judgment and exhaustion, we distance ourselves from them so we can just "do" their care and not "be" their care.

Our approach towards those in our care is directly influenced by how we perceive them. Changing the quality of the thoughts will change the quality of the experience. We like to think we are not judgmental, especially since we are in the helping profession. However, we judge ourselves and others all the time. It's common for healthcare workers to believe they're not judging a patient and, at the same time, experience feelings of frustration and thoughts that the patient is manipulating them—the same patients they claim to understand are suffering from an illness. I have heard caregivers say that they understand the myths associated with depression. One myth is that the patient can just "snap out of it." We may intellectualize and realize that depressed patients cannot snap out of it, yet most of us have admitted to feeling frustrated and discouraged that our patients aren't able to "pull up their socks" in a depression and "snap out of it." We may have even said statements like the following to a patient: "You should be happy; you just had a visit from your son; the sun is shining and you are having your favorite meal."

What we say, do and think are sometimes different things. Mahatma Gandhi echoed this sentiment when he said, "Happiness is when what you think, what you say and what you do are in harmony." I believe incongruence is a prime cause of our stress and one of our main hurdles in helping our patients. We say one thing yet think or feel other things. That is why it is so important to ask ourselves questions such as, "Are we part of the healing process or part of the dis-ease (lack of ease)?" Are we inadvertently creating more unease within ourselves and others by how we see the patient and the situation?

What we do in any given situation will depend on how we view the situation, where our first judgment occurs. This does not mean that we are uncaring, unfeeling helpers. In fact, it's just the opposite. The sensitivity, compassion and caring—the flame that brought us into this work—can be the very things that extinguish our fire. This is the fine line that we walk. That's why it's so important to find ways to look after ourselves and give to others at the same time. The caring must start with us. We have to find value in what we do. We have to find compassion for ourselves. We cannot give compassion unless we accept and have compassion for ourselves. Compassion feeds the soul of the giver and the receiver.

There may be many times in our helping journey when we can't cure or eliminate problems. Most caregivers working in long-term care or palliative situations have to focus on finding meaning in their work other than curing. Focusing on what we *can* do instead of what we can't do becomes vital for us when we feel helpless. Even though we might not experience the outcome we wish for, it is enough that we provide compassion and kindness. In sharing our compassion with others, we allow our true essence to shine through and feel the reward internally, as opposed to externally. Of course, it is always nice to hear that we're doing a good job and be compensated accordingly. It is great to know that we are appreciated, yet we don't usually hear this from the very ill or so-called "demanding" patients. We must come to the realization within ourselves that what we are *doing* and how we are *being* are vitally important. Are we *being* compassionate, patient and kind?

Can we truly experience a world without labels and judgments and accept ourselves and patients as they are? Can we recognize when our labels and judgments don't serve us or our patients well?

I like to think we can.

Questions to Ponder

- What do you really believe/think about this patient?
- What did you see?
- What did you think?
- What did you feel?
- What kind of reaction does this patient cause in you?
- What action do you take?

6

"DIFFICULT" PATIENTS

"It's not them, it's you.
It's not there, it's here.
It's not then, it's now."

—Author Unknown

Ah, the "difficult" patient. We all have stories of these types of patients. One caregiver shared with me her frustration with a particular resident. It was so worrisome that it kept her awake at night; she dreaded returning to her shift the next day. As caregivers, we can probably all relate to the dread associated with those we must look after for a shift, and the hope that we will get the "nice, sweet one."

She was a very pleasant caregiver, with a kind and thoughtful face. No one would have ever known that she was having difficulty with one particular resident. She "kept her cards close to her heart" and in so doing, was suffering numerous physical symptoms such as a cold that wouldn't go away and gastro-intestinal difficulties. Her sick days increased.

She shared that one resident in particular was very difficult to take care of. She felt that it wouldn't matter what she did since she was unable to provide any comfort or ease her distress. This particular patient would ring the bell continually.

"I dread going to work and answering Edna's bell," she confessed.

When she answered the bell, the patient would claim that she was "afraid and lonely" or complain that something wasn't right. The caregiver would explain that she didn't have a lot of time to spend with this anxious, demanding women and that she had twenty other residents to get up, bath and attend to.

When I asked her to identify the first thoughts that went through her mind when she thought about attending to this woman, she stated, "Frustration and helplessness."

I explained that those were feelings, not thoughts, and encouraged her to try identifying the possible thoughts that had created the feelings. (When we have strong emotional reactions, we go into our feelings right away and have difficulty identifying the thoughts that govern those feelings.)

The caregiver paused for a few moments to ponder the question then responded in a quiet voice, "Here she goes again. Another miserable day for the both of us."

I asked her how much she thought those types of thoughts would influence her ability to interact with the resident.

She hesitated once again and said, "A lot," but then added, "How can I not have those thoughts? They are true and all I know. I have never had a pleasant interaction with her."

I told her I believed that to be true and asked her if she wanted to look at ways to have a different type of interaction.

She responded, "Of course I want to."

I explained that there was incredible power in our thoughts. What we tell ourselves or don't tell ourselves becomes paramount in any interaction. I also explained that the thoughts she presently was experiencing were not serving her well and encouraged her to try having other thoughts and ideas that may serve her and her resident better.

Again she repeated that these thoughts were true (Ego was rearing its head!) She finally agreed to try to think of positive thoughts to replace the negatives ones before coming to work. We explored various thoughts that might lead to a different interaction with the patient. She came up with, "I wonder why she would act like this?"

All of sudden, there was interest in who this person was. She had become more than a label or her behavior. Could this one, simple thought become the catalyst for a different type of interaction?

Author Steven Covey seemed to think so when he said, "Seek first to understand then to be understood."

The caregiver was to try this new positive, inquiring, appreciative approach and then let me know how it was going. She came to one of our discussion groups with a big smile on her face and a bounce in her walk.

"Well, you're not going to believe this because I don't really believe this," she began, "but I am looking forward to seeing Edna."

I asked her what had changed.

"I guess I have changed, or at least my thoughts have. Before I spent so much time wishing and hoping she wouldn't ring that bell to bother me. Now when the bell rings, I search deeper to see what is going on instead of making it go away. It became about what's going on instead of trying to make it go away." She added in an excited voice to the rest of the participants, "Did you know she was in a concentration camp and was buried alive? No wonder she worries."

The best part of this story is that the caregiver was willing to do something different to make things better. So much wisdom is gained when we listen to others. I often share and repeat what this caregiver said in regard to how she saw her patient situation now. The caregiver's words deserve to be repeated again:

It became what's was going on and not trying to make it go away.

We are each other's greatest teachers. How many times in our career do we wish things were different and spend enormous amounts of energy wanting things to be different? Accepting our patients as they are and changing our outlook and approach to them can be very freeing.

Dr. Carl Rodger, the guru of the compassionate approach, coined "Unconditional positive regard." This is a deep knowing that we are accepted, no matter what—understanding that we will be helped in our situation and not be judged by what we do or don't do. This open, nonjudgmental approach is the glue that can hold a healing relationship together, especially when working with difficult patients.

Questions to Ponder

- What do you do when you encounter a difficult patient or resident?
- Are you judgmental?
- Do you label?
- Do you avoid?
- Minimize contact?

- Are you short, brief, sterile; in and out as quickly as possible?
- Do you go back to your colleagues and complain that, "such and such are a miserable ---? This is a thankless job."

What makes a patient challenging or difficult?

Difficult patients have been defined as "patients who are medically challenging, interpersonally difficult, psychiatrically ill, chronically medically ill, or lacking in social support" (Adams & Murray).

This description could just about cover everyone, so it might be helpful to better understand ourselves and the so-called "difficult" people. It is easy to have amazing magic moments with the so-called "sweet, likeable" patients, however, these aren't the ones who are likely to extinguish our flame of compassion. Why do some people we help (or try to help) bother us more that others?

The Swiss psychiatrist and one of the founding fathers of psychology, Carl Jung, stated, "Everything that irritates us about others can lead us to an understanding of ourselves." He also stated that "the meeting of two personalities is like the contact of two chemical substances; if there is any reaction, both are transformed."

I believe difficult patients cause "allergic reactions" in us. In Dale Larson's book, *The Helper's Journey*, psychologist Norman Kagan refers to the term "interpersonal allergies." This is described as "our usually unconscious response to stimuli that triggers a physically and emotionally sensitive reaction." It is a reaction we can all relate to at any given time in our helping life—when we get stretched beyond the point of wanting to make a connection with some patients. In these situations, we usually want to provide just the minimal amount of care, get in and out quickly and try to avoid eye contact (this only encourages the undesirable annoying behavior). If their door is open, we look straight ahead and increase our pace so they don't see us pass by. Sound familiar?

Difficult patients challenge a healthcare worker's sense of competence, self- confidence and skills. It triggers an interpersonal allergy involving frustration and helplessness. Usually the difficult patients have been described as angry, loud, demanding, controlling, complaining, unappreciative, aggressive, manipulative, rambling, annoying, and verbally and physically abusive. Usually, these patients are difficult to communicate with, exaggerate their symptoms, and have incongruent, unrealistic expectations. Lorne Ladner, psychologist and author of the book *The Lost Art of Compassion* said, "Often it is the difficult people who are suffering the most intensely and who are therefore in most need of compassion."

On politically correct days, patients who test our egos to the max are referred to as "difficult" or "challenging." On the not-so-politically correct days, they are labeled, "pains in the butt." Neither of these comments acknowledges the humanness of the difficult encounter, because what accompanies the humanness is anger, resentment, fear and anguish—emotions that are difficult for most caring staff to contend with.

Our goal is to be all right with these emotions and understand that this is the core essence of a difficult patient.

Questions to ponder

- Do you have a difficult patient, resident or family story?
- What makes them difficult for you?
- Do you seem to be having more than your share of "difficult" situations"? What could be the cause of this?

- How do you usually cope with difficult patient situations?
- How can our difficult patients be our greatest teachers?

7

OUR PERCEPTIONS-
WHAT DO WE SEE?

"Your assumptions are your windows of the world.
Scrub them off every once and awhile or
the light won't come in."

—ALAN ALDA

Bob and the nursing staff were at odds. The stroke he had suffered was affecting his ability to communicate, leaving him feeling angry and frustrated. One evening when the lights were turned down low, Bob sat in a Broda chair hollering, screaming and yelling continually. He was miserable.

Diane, the caregiver, decided to pull up a chair and try to make conversation. She decided to use a different approach. Instead of telling him everything would get better, she took a moment to think about how he might be feeling at this point in his life. She surmised that he probably felt isolated and alone and that no one wanted to take the time to know him.

Diane decided to be honest with him. "Bob, you can yell and scream as loud and as long as you want," she said.

Bob stopped and looked at her, waiting to hear more. She told him that she knew he hated the place and that he wanted to leave, and admitted that she would, too, if she were in his position. Diane continued to empathize with Bob's feelings and acknowledge that he was having a hard time expressing himself. Diane apologized to Bob and said, "I know you hate the Broda chair you are in right now, and if you want out, just give me the thumbs up"

Two thumbs immediately popped up. She asked him if it would be alright if she put him back in bed. He immediately gave another "thumbs up" and a grunt. She apologized again for being a pain in the butt (interesting to note most staff saw *him* as a pain in the butt) and he laughed and smiled with Diane. They laughed for ten minutes straight.

She shared this story with other staff, and soon all the staff was looking for his smile and thumbs up. Bob passed away a few months ago, and staff still go by his room, claiming they miss his smile and thumbs up. As Diane, the healthcare worker said, "You don't realize when you give some of yourself to a resident how much has been given to you."

I believe we all have similar stories yet don't always focus on them or share them with others. No doubt, there are people we are working with right now who can help us bring out these feelings, if we are open and willing to focus on the positive. Or, even better, we can be the ones to light the way for other caregivers. Of course, there will always be dark and difficult days, however, you can ease this burden by remembering to look for beauty and light in the simplest of actions.

She was new to the unit, yet not to care-giving. She had been a nurse for over twenty-five years. This unit had very difficult, agitated, aggressive Alzheimer's patients. One patient in particular was causing the staff a lot of distress, frustration and tension. This new nurse informed the staff that she would like to try music to ease his suffering and agitation. The rest of the team was quick to respond, "That has been tried many times and it is useless. We need to up his PRN medication."

She said, "I would like to try anyway" She started with big band music then old-time music, rock, and finally classical.

The staff again approached her and said, "We told you he is beyond help with music at this stage of his disease."

Still undaunted, she went home and the next day brought back a CD of animal noises and sounds from nature. This CD soothed him, and the staff was grateful and quick to borrow it on each of their shifts. Some of them commented, "Now we have a solution that works."

The caregiver replied quietly, "For now."

I love this story and the discussion that took place amongst the staff. Everyone wanted to do something. No one wanted to see this man in distress. What makes one person persist when everything and everyone is telling her it will be in vain? How can we all look at situations with fresh eyes and perspective? I especially loved her last comment: "For now." So much of how we think is in absolutes, and we want guarantees and permanent fixes. Saying, "For now," illustrates how important *now* is. This moment, this time.

One facility had a resident with dementia following a stroke. As a result, he had difficulty communicating. He would continually throw himself on the floor throughout the day. This was most upsetting to staff and other visitors. Some staff believed he was trying to get them in trouble with his family and management and accuse them of "bad care." Other staff believed he really didn't know what he was doing and picked him up immediately, which resulted in an aggressive outburst by the resident. Light was finally shone on the case when the staff felt comfortable approaching the family and sharing their challenges with them.

"Dad always liked lying on the floor. That was where he composed his music," the family told them.

He was a composer! He liked the floor! As Anais Nin, writer and diarist, said, "We don't always see the world as it is, we see it as we are."

Our power lies in the ability to change how we see the situation, which then changes how we think, feel and react. We spend a large part of our day in reaction mode, where we don't believe we have the time to pause and see what is causing our reaction. As a result, we find ourselves in a volatile situation.

Questions to Ponder

- Do you recognize your inner critic? What does it say? What does it tell you? How does your ego influence you interactions?
- Do you ever pause during a shift and actually reflect on what you are seeing, doing, thinking and feeling?
- Can you recognize your ego in healthcare?
- What is your ego saying to you?

MAGIC MOMENT MODES

8

ACKNOWLEDGEMENT

"I long to accomplish a great and noble task,
but it is my chief duty to accomplish small
tasks as if they were great and noble."

—HELEN KELLER

Now that we have identified the hurdles of helping, we will now focus on the "modes" of magic moments. (A mode is "a way, a tool, a method, an approach and a practice.")

It is not easy to create meaningful opportunities or "spaces" in our workday, where we are absolutely, consciously, compassionately present in the moment with our patients. We get used to accepting things the "way they are," and it takes courage and desire to determine if there is another way. Even more difficult is recognizing that these spaces, when created, will help us find meaning in work. It is important for us to honor the need to create these spaces and to find tremendous value in doing so.

The first step in creating magic moments is to acknowledge the need to do so. Acknowledgement comes from the word "recognition," which involves "existence, authority, truth or genuineness." The term "to recognize" comes from the Latin term *recognoscere*, which means "recall to mind; know again; examine." The phrase "to know again" is very powerful, as it gently reminds us why we as helpers do the work we do. The Oxford dictionary defines acknowledgement as, "agreeing to the truth, admitting, owning, noticing, validating, and recognize the events and situations in our life." Acknowledging where we are in our helping journey and questioning if we are functioning in "survivor shift mode" during our shift or actually thriving in our work becomes paramount. Acknowledging where we are as helper is not an easy thing to do, as it requires deep personal reflection and valuing the time it takes to do so. Webster's dictionary states that acknowledgement is "the act of recognizing, in particular, relationships." To us caregivers, this means noticing and examining with genuineness our helping roles and relationships and exploring what it would take to enhance those relationships.

Acknowledging ourselves and our role as healthcare workers, as well as acknowledging patients with all their fears, worries concerns and behaviors, is an essential first step in the Magic Moments modes. I had never really thought about how I saw my role as a healthcare professional. I realize now how imperative and refreshing it is to take some time to reflect on how I see my role and how I am currently providing care. I now understand that it does not serve me to focus on feelings of inadequacy. I have learned to simply acknowledge and observe these feelings and reactions and not become attached to them. Even though I may experience these feelings, they do not define me.

Acknowledgment is a two-step process. First, we need to acknowledge that we want (and need) to do things differently and be different. Second, we need to value our acknowledgment of patients in order to create the magic. With acknowledgement come awareness and a desire to see the potential in a situation instead of only the deficits. We know where we are and have a desire to create something more and look at ways to thrive in our work. If we are on the work-a-day track, it is important to get off and take a look and check out if we're headed in the right direction. If we don't get off once in awhile, we risk being hit by a train coming in the opposite direction or being overtaken by another train that deems us too slow or becoming the train and running over everyone in our path. Only by stepping aside and taking a look at the situation will we be able to identify, create and focus on the positive moments so we can create that all-important magic in our work.

The joy of being in the magic moment is not about thinking; it is about being consciously present in that moment. When we are present every moment, every task is performed with deliberation and design, rich with depth and meaning. I call this *M.O.D.E.*: Moments Of Design Every time. We are co-creators in every moment. Whatever we bring into the moment, we will create. If we are in reactive, automatic, unconscious mode, we will usually have negative, anxious and depreciative results. If we offer patience, understanding, openness, acceptance and a sense of humor, the results will be much different! The choice is ours.

One of our choices may be to acknowledge that we need to rekindle the magic in our work. Another choice may be to put in the effort to do this. If we are satisfied with our current status and hurdles in helping, we probably won't want to go further with this. If we are satisfied we probably wouldn't be reading this book in the first place. Deep down inside, we know that there is more to our work than what we are doing and that "things" are just getting in the way. We somehow have to acknowledge and honor the work we do. We aren't just "putting in time." We are creating our role, moment to moment, in the way we interact with our patients.

It is helpful to acknowledge how we see our role in healthcare and consciously decide what role we want to create in our work. According to Rachel Remen, M.D., Clinical Professor of Family and Community Medicine at the UCSF School of Medicine, "… our roles as caregivers are really a reflection of how we see life." Dr. Remen, states that "when you help, you see life as weak; when you fix, you see life as broken; and when you serve, you see life as whole. When we serve in this way, we understand that each person's suffering is also my suffering, that their joy is also my joy, and then the impulse to serve arises naturally—our natural wisdom and compassion presents itself quite simply. A server knows that they're being used and has the willingness to be used in the service of something greater. We may help or fix many things in our lives, but when we serve, we are always in the service of wholeness."

It really is about finding meaning and wholeness in our work. There will be days that magic modes will be tested and there will be times when our old baggage will resurface, causing us to feel incapacitated in our work. It is essential that we be tenacious, get rid of expectations, let go, honor thy self, and welcome the difficult days.

It is usually on difficult days that we question the meaning of our work. During these times, we should gently remind ourselves that the magic is always there, even when it's difficult to find.

It will be up to us to continue to acknowledge, honor and appreciate the profoundness in the magic of moments and look for ways to accentuate the "ahh" moments.

Acknowledging our patients is a powerful Magic moment's tool. We can transform our relationships with our patients when we are interested and concerned about them. Greet each patient as a holy encounter. "I vow to give my full attention to his or her needs today." What are you acknowledging and paying attention to today? What is taking up your energy and concern? Is it the patients needs or the difficulties of the day? Philosopher and humanist Jose Ortega Gasset said, "Tell me what you pay attention to and I will tell you who you are."

Use the magic moment mode of acknowledgement as a daily tool. It is important to keep our mind focused on individual needs and not let ourselves be distracted by past or future thoughts that can take us out of the moment, e.g., *It is already 10:00 AM and I have to get Mr. Smith fed and bathed.*

Viewing Exercise

- ✓ Spend one day writing down what you observed today.
- ✓ Notice what you see, think, and feel and how you react to the situations you find yourself in. This will give you a clear picture of what you focus your attention on during the day.

Questions to Ponder

- • How do you see your role?
- • How do you see the work you do?
- • Do you see yourself as a fixer, helper, curer, healer, server?

What are we missing?

In our rush to get our jobs done, we tend to focus on the future and past and avoid the present moment. "The present is holy ground," author Alfred North Whitehead said. Magic Moments involve honoring the present and paying attention to every moment.

For five or more years, Beth, a manager of a long-term care unit, had one-sided discussions with one particular resident, who was in a wheelchair. Just before she'd leave the unit, she would tell the resident, whose name was Albert, that she was going home to cook supper for her family. Sometimes she would even share what she was going to make. For months he never acknowledged or responded to her comments, except once. That day, she had had a very bad day and was feeling harried. When she rushed by Albert, he yelled out, "Hey, hey, what are you going to make for supper tonight?" Until that moment, Beth had no idea how much her so-called "one- sided" discussions had meant to that individual.

In my caregiver wellness workshop I encourage participants to really notice what is going on around them and to pay attention to the possibility of what they could be missing and not acknowledging during their shift. One particular caregiver who had taken this advice was surprised by what she had been missing. It was a cold dreary day in the middle of winter and she noticed one chickadee, then another and then hundreds of them. She marveled that they had likely always been there in that concrete jungle, however, in her rush she had never noticed them. (The chickadee is a wonderful metaphor for acknowledging resiliency, cheer and courage, as these are the birds I hear singing when the temperature is -40C!)

In our daily life, there is a constant flow of energy from us to others and back again. The words and thoughts we use influence this energy flow. The words we use define our reality and what is important to us. Some words and phrases can actually take us out of the present and make us feel powerless. Words like *if only, could have, should have, would have, will be, must be, but, going to, assume that* lower our energy and remove us from the present, whereas words like *I am, I am here, I am open, I am compassionate, I am courageous, I am patient* are powerful, high energy words that keep us in the present.

The Simple Things

The simplest, smallest gestures from the heart often have the most profound impact on those we serve. It's not always important how many technical skills we have or how many procedures we can do—if they are not delivered with warmth and compassion, everything becomes cold, sterile and dark. Researchers from the Nashville Tennessee Vanderbilt School of Medicine indicate that physicians who are most likely to be sued by their patients are not only inept but are deemed uncompassionate, uncaring with poor interpersonal skills.

Mary, an emergency physician, said how annoying and frustrated she used to feel when a patient asked for a glass of water or facecloth. She was prepared to do a tracheotomy or intubation but much too busy for the "little things." It wasn't until she was admitted to the hospital with a life-threatening illness that she realized how precious these little things were and how much of a difference they made to a patient's comfort. She was embarrassed to confess that she would ask for little things such as a blanket or to have someone check a tube when she was in bed because she "just wanted to see someone." After this experience, she is now quick to bring that blanket or other little thing to provide comfort and demonstrate her compassion.

Recently, I saw a colleague at one of our health facilities. She appeared fatigued, in pain, and was being pushed in a wheelchair by her husband. I spoke with her for a few minutes and told her about the book I was writing. She claimed she should write a book called "On the other side." She explained it truly was the little moments of acknowledgment that mattered and how often she had underestimated that in her nursing career. She shared how frustrated she had been while trying to read a get-well message. She rang the bell for help, only to be on the abrupt end of a frustrated caregiver who lectured her that she had more important things to do than bring her cards closer to her. An opportunity for kindness had flown out the window, and the nurse, who was now the patient, was given precious insight into "the other side."

Last year my son was in for a "routine" tonsillectomy. (While this may be routine for the medical staff, it is never routine for the parents and the children. Anytime parents must leave their beloved children in the hands of another, it is a frightening experience.) We had been waiting for some time to take our son up to another floor for surgery. We could see how busy it was, as staff members rushed by us. Finally, we were told to follow a person up the stairs and wait. When we did, we found ourselves in the middle of another busy hallway. We hoped someone would notice that we were sitting there and perhaps smile or give us a word of encouragement. Suddenly, a nurse who had nothing to do with our surgery stopped and acknowledged my son, husband and me. She gave us a warm "I see you" smile. She even checked to see how much longer we would have to wait for the anesthetist. Ten hours later, my son commented on how nice it was of that nurse to stop and talk to us. Somehow, that very busy nurse had found time to acknowledge us and in so doing, we were able to experience her compassion and sensitivity. Why did she do that, when so many others passed us by? Rabbi Dov Baer of Mezritch says, "When you gaze at an object you bring blessing to it." We were most certainly blessed in that hallway!

One Good Word

My Mom was recently in the hospital for a knee replacement and, knowing I was writing this book, made some very good observations. She claimed to have developed a very comforting relationship with a student nurse. When I asked her what made him comforting, she explained, "It wasn't that he had a lot of time to spend with me—he didn't—but when he was beside me, he would hold my hand and look at me and tell me what he was doing. I especially liked that when he entered my room, he would always say, "Hello, Mrs. Helga, it's Jason." When my Mom told Jason's supervising nurse how good he was, the supervisor's abrupt response was, "It was about time he got it."

Too many times we hear good things about another staff member and fail to pass on this important feedback or feel pride as a team—sometimes may even feel slighted (What about me?) It is important to acknowledge the good work of our colleagues.

My mom went on to say that she shared a room with another elderly woman who was recovering from hip surgery. "Maybe she was a bit crabby and abrupt with the nurse," she said. "I think she was really suffering and in a lot of a pain. Anyway, she was probably hard on the staff because of her suffering. We all cope differently, you know, and, well, the staff was in and out of her bedside in a flash. They spent more time with me. I think it was because your mother is just so sweet," my mother added quietly with a big smile.

We had a chuckle and I was once again reminded of our humanness as caregivers and how difficult it is to be there for someone who is not easy to be around. If we don't find ways to help ourselves in these difficult situations, we only cause ourselves and our patients more grief. We lose ourselves and our purpose as helpers, and they lose out on our healing, compassionate presence.

9

KINDNESS AND COMPASSION

"The greatest reward for serving others is the satisfaction in your own heart."

—Unknown

Kindness and compassion are pivotal aspects of our work, however, there are times when our "kindness factor" becomes depleted. The truth is, caregivers are usually unkind to themselves, in thought and deed. We tell ourselves that we aren't good enough or we can't take that well- deserved break because we are much too busy—despite knowing that if we miss our break, we won't be there in spirit. But it is with our spirit that we connect with patients. Without that, we are mere shells and unable to make the connections that we truly long for, especially with our more difficult patients. We must first be true to ourselves and take time for ourselves. We need to find and create kind moments for ourselves at work. We must take time to go to the bathroom when we get the urge, splurge on that chocolate chip cookie in the cafeteria, or find a quiet space when we need it. We mustn't forget to tell ourselves that we are doing a good job or to find that one person, be it staff or patient, who will rejuvenate us. (More self-renewal concepts will be discussed in chapter 13.) We must remind ourselves why we chose this work in the first place. (Yes, we did, in fact, choose it!) Then we must try not to be so overwhelmed that we deprive ourselves from our greatest gift—reaching out and connecting with people when they are the most vulnerable. If we are open, we can learn from all patients in our care, even the most difficult ones.

Giving and Receiving

There are two types of relationships: consumptive and generative. Consumptive relationships generally refer to those relationships where we feel drained and lacking in energy. In those relationships we may feel like we are always giving and that someone always needs something from us. In generative relationships we feel an energy exchange and possibly a refueling of energy.

Our role as helpers usually falls in the realm of consumptive—or at least we have a tendency to focus on the "needing" aspect. We helpers are notorious for attracting people in our life who always "need" something. In fact, if we aren't careful, we end up measuring our self-worth by these types of relationships. But we can only give so much before we must receive in order to restore ourselves. We do not always acknowledge that we must also receive in our role as compassionate servers, or that we need relationships with people who energize and revitalize us.

Giving should not define who we are. I admit that it is not always easy to receive. I have never found it easy. If someone assists me or does something kind for me, I immediately ask myself what I can do to pay them back or start to feel inadequate and guilty that I had to ask for help. I am now more conscious of these thought processes and am practicing to receive the gift of kindness from others. I am also practicing to receive and bask in the glow of compassion for myself. I am becoming much more aware that at any given moment I can give compassion to myself and those in my care and receive compassion and care from others. In "generative" relationships we feel reciprocity—giving and receiving. We can incorporate this in our role as helpers so that when we give, there is something to receive, if and when we are open to it.

Helping relationships tend to be consumptive but they don't have to be. Being aware of who we spend our time with outside of work is important. If we are a parent or a caregiver outside work, it's all the more reason to spend time with those who can give to us, or to participate in activities that refuel us. (We will look at this more closely in the self-care section of the book.) Developing an awareness of our ability to receive while we serve others is fundamental to our ability to show kindness and compassion, and it must start with ourselves.

A student of Zen once asked the Abbot what it meant to serve others.

"What others? Serve yourself!" the Abbot responded.

"How do I serve myself?" the student persisted.

"Take care of others," was the Abbot's reply.

According to Naomi Levy, author of the book *To Begin Again*, "Visiting someone who is ill takes away 1/60th of the person's illness." The ancient sages realized that being in the presence of another kind, compassionate human being can lift a person up. Lifting up someone else is a way of lifting up ourselves. It is a fascinating exchange of energy. Take a moment to think of a helping situation where you have experienced this pure potential "goose bump" experience and said, "Yes, this is why I do this work!"

In our search for compassion, it is crucial to be aware of our feelings and reactions. There are basically three different types of feelings we experience as we go through life: pleasant, unpleasant and neutral. It's not the feelings themselves that cause problems for us; it's how we *react* to these feelings. Being aware of and acknowledging our feelings will help to prevent us from getting caught up in the drama of our reactions. If, for example, a patient really irritates you, say, "Hey, this patient really irritates me." Then let go of the irritation, dig deep to find what is causing your irritation and search for the humanness of the encounter. Most likely, you'll discover that your attachments, expectations, labels and judgments (ego) are the culprits. Be a conscious observer of your feelings and reactions. Watch them move through you like a cloud in a sky and be replaced by a sense of wonder and acceptance.

According to Lorne Ladner, "Even-mindedness is key to developing strong compassion. Even-mindedness is not about indifference and not caring; it is about relationships free of attachments, aversions. It is about being aware of and 'knowing.' "

Questions to Ponder

- How do you find compassion for yourself?
- How do you show compassion for yourself?
- What does compassion and kindness in your work as a healthcare professional mean to you?
- How do you show compassion in your work as a healthcare professional?
- What would prevent you from showing compassion?
- What happens when you do not show compassion to yourself or your patients?

Separated but Connected

For protection, caregivers separate themselves from their patients. While this separation hinders us in our work, we fear that without this separation, we may become enmeshed with our patients and no longer able to function in a healthy way. Our challenge is to find that neutral place in the middle where the separation is blurred; where we are able to feel our patients' pain without taking it on ourselves. We all have this innate ability, as well as our own unique way of serving those in our care. Be on the lookout for moments when the separation between you and another individual disappears. Remember, it's not about taking on a patient's difficulties; it's about experiencing a special connection with another human being, and knowing that this is their journey and our role is to just "be" there with them.

Edith Stein, philosopher of empathy, explained that helping professionals need not lose their therapeutic objectivity, as so many fear, in getting "too close" to their patients. Instead, what is experienced is a kind of holistic listening that can unite the helper with the patient, yet allow them to remain fully separate in the healing process. It is in identification alone that we lose our objectivity and become destructively fused with the patient.

According to Dr. Rachel Remen, "Professionalism has embedded in service a sense of difference, a certain distance. But on the deepest level, service is an experience of belonging, an experience of connection to others and to the world around us. It is this connection that gives us the power to bless the life in others. Without it, the life in them would not respond to us."

An old Rabbi once asked his pupils how they could tell when the night had ended and the day had begun.

"Could it be," asked one of the students, "when you can see an animal in the distance and tell whether it's a sheep or a dog?"

"No," answered the Rabbi.

"Is it when you can look at a tree in the distance and tell whether it's a fig tree or a peach tree?" another asked.

"No," answered the Rabbi.

"Then what is it?" the pupils demanded.

"It is when you can look on the face of any man or woman and see that it is your sister or brother. Because if you cannot see this, it is still night."

Somewhere along the way, we may have forgotten that we possess the power to comfort another human being. I believe that our work-a-day lives are filled with many opportunities to bless and nurture others, yet we have become so medically minded and cure minded that we often ignore opportunities to just bring peace and compassion to a tormented soul. We minimize the effect that our interactions with an individual will have and believe that no matter what we say or do, we will have little or no effect on their healing. However, healing is not about curing; it about restoring the essence of what it means to be human. Knowing that someone truly cares about you and is there for you can be the best balm in the world!

How can we be there for someone when we're running on empty? The times when we think we have no more to give are the times we need to give tenderness, patience and a gentle smile. When we believe we can't possibly be compassionate or speak lovingly to someone and then consciously give the very thing we think we don't have (a smile, kind word or comforting touch), all of a sudden we start to receive! Our impatience and irritation miraculously begin to melt away and are replaced by warm feelings deep in our soul.

Arthur Jersild, a developmental psychologist and author, said, "Compassion is the ultimate and most meaningful embodiment of emotional maturity. It is through compassion that a person achieves the highest peak and the deepest reach in his or her search for self-fulfillment."

The other day I entered a fast food chain with three hungry children and a long line. I observed the tension, from both the staff and the patrons in the lineup. No one was smiling. I found myself becoming very irritable and impatient. I noticed the staff also seemed irritated and rude and believed they didn't like or care about their job or the patrons' time. I found myself eagerly anticipating my arrival at the counter so I could give them a "piece of my mind." At the same time, I consciously decided that I didn't like the feelings associated with these thoughts and the situation. Even though it was the last thing I thought I wanted or needed to do, I forced myself to smile, cajole and appreciate the work the staff was doing. The result was incredible! The one staff member I deemed the most thoughtless and cold gave me the biggest smile that went right to my core. One smile and then another joke began to transform the entire experience for those who were willing to engage in this positive energy and leave the negative energy behind.

I encourage you to try this for yourself. If you encounter someone at home or work that you don't want to smile at or talk kindly to, force yourself to do the very thing you believe you are unable to do and see what happens. Do you feel a release, acceptance and openness? Chances are, if you thought that person was hurting, tired, lost, afraid or alone, you were likely feeling and experiencing the same thing. As caregivers, we carry a lot of emotional burdens, which can develop into ailments that can take a toll on our psychological and physical wellbeing. It is in our best interests to develop ways to let go and let be. During stressful times, it is especially important to surround ourselves with people we know are able to give back to us. We need a reservoir of compassion in our work and many places where we can reflect and refuel so we can continue to provide compassionate care to our patients.

"Tibetan metaphor for compassion consists of many small puddles that can evaporate more easy than a deep expansive long last reservoir," according to Lorne Ladner.

Two monks were traveling together. One monk was more senior and the other a novice. They ended up beside a river where a woman was in need of help to cross the river. The senior monk decided that they should both help carry the woman across the river. The novice monk reminded him that it was unacceptable to touch a woman, let alone carry her. The senior monk convinced the novice monk that this was what they needed to do, and they did carry the women across the river. The woman was very grateful. An hour or so later, the novice monk was still disturbed by the notion of carrying the woman

"We should never have carried the woman," he said. "It was wrong."

The senior monk looked up with a big bright smile and said, "I left her by the shore, but you are still carrying her."

The Difficult Patient

We are all familiar with the angst we feel before entering a "difficult" patient's room. Thoughts of the yelling, swearing and condemning remarks that will likely ensue make it a challenge, to say the least. Most healthcare professionals can relate to walking by "difficult" patients' rooms quickly and being extremely careful to avoid eye contact with them. This is usually related to fear of aggravating or encouraging them and wanting to avoid the patient and their undesirable behavior. In most cases, we want to avoid contact with someone we perceive to be difficult because we don't know how to respond positively to the patient. In my experience, the best way to respond to a difficult patient is to develop compassion for that patient—that is, let go of my own hurt, anger, frustration and prejudice and suffering, and see the patient as a person who is suffering. While it may be incredibly challenging to provide compassionate, nonjudgmental care to a difficult patient, doing so is not only crucial to our helping relationships but vital for creating and honoring the magic moments in our work.

Fortunately, not all your colleagues will view your "difficult" patients the same way you do. Another staff member might find him or her quite pleasant and endearing. When I encounter a difficult patient, I find it helpful to ask if there is anyone who does not have trouble with that patient. Usually, at least one staff member responds. I then encourage this staff member to share his or her thoughts, ideas and approaches in regard to delivering care to this difficult patient. If other staff members are open and willing, there is enormous learning for all. Author and poet Ralph Waldo Emerson says it well: "In every person there is something wherein I may learn and in that I am his pupil."

One powerful way humans show compassion is through touch. A gentle touch can go a long way to ease and comfort a person. This might mean a handshake, an arm around the shoulders or a pat on the hand. (Of course, we must always be sensitive to the patient's comfort.) In Zur and Nordmarken's article "To Touch or Not to Touch: Exploring the Myth of Prohibition on Touch in Psychotherapy and Counseling," touch has long been regarded as having qualities to ease and heal: "The medicinal aspect of touch has been known and utilized since earliest recorded medical history, 25 centuries ago. Touch unleashes a stream of healing chemical responses including a decrease in stress hormones and an increase in serotonin and dopamine levels. Touch increases the immune system's cytotoxic capacity thereby helping our body maintain its defenses. Massage has been shown to decrease anxiety, depression, hyperactivity, inattention, stress hormones and cortisol levels."

Mrs. Smith was the type of resident that all staff wanted to avoid. She was in a wheelchair and was physically and verbally abusive. The staff never knew when they'd be the brunt of her anger and aggression. While they could empathize and understand that her illness was causing these behaviors, for the most part the person got lost in all her disturbing behaviors. We talked about what we could do differently with these types of encounters.

One healthcare worker named Elsie decided that in the following weeks she would make the extra effort to try to have a "moment" with the resident. Other staff members quickly informed Elsie that it was a waste of time or would take up too much time and that she could end up getting hurt. Elsie swallowed the lump in her throat and approached the resident cautiously. The resident's first response was "What the hell do you want now?"

Elsie looked at the resident intently and responded, "I am just checking to see if you are okay."

The resident became quiet and said in a soft voice, "Would you listen to me?" Then she went on to explain that she missed her home and her dad. Rather than replying with the common response, "This is your home now," Elsie asked her to tell her more about her home and her father. The resident's eyes glazed over with unshed tears that fell in droplets down her cheeks. The resident allowed Elsie to comfort her by wrapping her arm around her shoulders. They even shared a smile and a laugh amongst the tears.

Elsie described this encounter as one of her most amazing experiences and would later reflect on and share it with other staff members. She realized that she may never have another magic encounter with that resident again, yet it encouraged her and others to continue to seek out other meaningful encounters. It also became a reminder that "finding meaning" can be as varied and unique as each person.

I have always been fascinated by the Pygmalion effect. The Pygmalion effect was described following the famous Broadway play in which a poor working girl showed that she could behave like a princess when she was treated like one, and taught carefully. This proves that how we treat someone greatly influences how they feel about themselves. Getting to know and understand our patients will not only pave the road for our compassion but foster a trusting, therapeutic "magic moments" relationship with them.

I agree with Sir William Osler, who says, "It is more important to know the person that has the disease than it is to know the disease that the person has."

A resident became aggressive during bathing and simply refused to be bathed in the morning. In that particular facility, bathing was scheduled in the morning at designated times throughout the week. One staff member decided to investigate this resident's personal history and found out that for thirty years of his life he had lived on the street, didn't get up until the afternoon and most likely bathed once a month. By acknowledging this resident's life story, the staff was able to shift how they saw the situation. He was no longer the defiant resident and became a person with a story.

Questions to Ponder

- Who is this person?
- Are they more then their paralysis and angry words?
- What do they hope for?
- What do they dream?
- What do they fear?
- What are their concerns and worries?
- What brings them comfort?
- What do they enjoy?
- What were they proficient at?
- What did they do for a living?
- What is important to them?
- Who is important to them?

Little Acts of Kindness

Contrary to what many might think, compassion has more to do with the small, conscious, everyday acts than the colossal epics. Over and over, when people describe compassionate acts, they refer not to monumental actions or events in their lives but to the simple, kind behaviors—ways of listening and supporting that are hard to describe because of their apparent mundaneness. How often do we downplay these little acts of compassion?

Compassion is such a large part of our work, yet we rarely talk about it. We are more apt to witness or provide compassion in our daily lives as healthcare workers without realizing the enormous potential to transform our helping relationships with it.

One day I acknowledged an act of compassion in a long-term care facility. I was in a hallway and a wheelchair-bound resident's blanket had fallen off. I observed a staff member stop in her tracks, put down what she was holding, tuck the blanket up close around the resident's neck and shoulders, give her a little squeeze and say, "There! I bet that is cozier." When I approached this staff member and acknowledged her act of sweet kindness, she shrugged it off and said, "It was no big deal. I was just doing my job." I disagree. She was doing much more than just "doing her job;" she was "being" with another person in a time of need.

Sometimes we may equate doing our job with our procedures, techniques and treatment and miss the pivotal component of kindness and compassion. In Julie Sladden's article "Does the Whole Health Care Need to be Filled Holistically?" Professor David Peters, clinical director of the University of Westminster's School of Integrated Health, believes there is conflict between target measure and compassion. "Compassion and imagination are too often forced to give way to targets and performance measures. So doctors and nurses are losing the confidence they once had that they made a difference to their patients. Some are even leaving the profession."

Wayne Muller, minister and author of *How Should I live,* describes kindness as "a seed; it is not an impressive thing. It is what can grow from the seed that is impressive." He stressed the importance of striking a balance between our inner growth and outer service.

Wayne Muller's questions for you to ponder:

1) Who am I?
2) What do I love?
3) How should I live knowing that I will die?
4) What is my gift to the family of the earth?

So often we do nothing because we believe that whatever we do will not be enough or will not change the complaining or ease the situation. We miss the opportunity of being there; with no other purpose than to just share a moment in time with kindness and compassion.

Exercise

- ✓ Describe the kindest person you know. It could be a mentor or someone from your past or present. It might be a hero-type or just someone you know. Describe the trait(s) this person has that demonstrate he/she is kind.

Key considerations regarding compassion and kindness

- We have to beware of others' thoughts and feelings and show concern and caring.
- Compassion does not have anything to do with heroic monumental tasks; rather compassion really involves the simple and ordinary.
- Compassion may be seen as less valuable then measurable technological performance basis procedures.
- Without compassion, healthcare professionals are more inclined to question the meaning in their work and whether they are making a difference.

10

YOUR LISTENING PRESENCE

*"Listening is an attitude of the heart,
a genuine desire to be with another
which both attracts and heals."*

—J. ISHAM

ARE WE LISTENING?

Most of us know the value of listening, yet how often do we truly listen? Are we giving someone our full presence and attention, or are we there in body only? Are we hearing what the person is saying, or are we thinking about what *we* will say? It's not that we don't want to listen or don't see the value in listening. We just find it difficult to tame our minds so we can be truly there for someone. Whether we realize it or not, our body language speaks volumes. Our gestures and eyes are powerful communicators. (Eyes really are "the window of the soul.") Listening is one of the most talked-about and least-adhered-to concepts. To truly listen, we must be fully present. This takes practice and a sincere desire to improve and create meaningful moments in your work. It also requires constant attention and awareness, as well as forgiveness and gentleness when we fall off track.

When we give someone our complete attention, it becomes a profound encounter. Author Joseph Rael, also described as a visionary, says, "The true human is someone who is aware, someone who is moment by moment, totally and completely merged with life. He is a listener. She is a listener. Out of that capacity of inner and outer listening comes the quality of humility. The true listener is no longer defined by desires or attachments. Instead, he or she is sensitized to consciousness."

Listening Exercise

- ✓ I don't like to listen to…..
- ✓ I like to listen to….
- ✓ I avoid listening to…..
- ✓ I could improve how well I listen to…
- ✓ I always listen to…
- ✓ I rarely listen to…

The following are paramount in developing listening skills:

- Showing genuine interest in the other person and encouraging him or her to talk
- Ensuring that your body language encourages the person who is speaking
- Smiling
- Making eye contact
- Nodding your head
- Your tone of voice
- Having an open, welcoming body position

- Being aware of thoughts and judgments that may come to mind
- Listening without anticipating what the patient is saying
- Avoiding judgment/planning what to say (this will go a long way to bridging the gap between you and your patient)
- Asking questions to clarify and encourage the patient to continue
- Remaining calm without being detached when a patient is in emotional distress

Listening to someone who is angry or in distress is not easy. It is difficult to be in the moment with someone without thinking ahead to what else needs to be done or how to respond to a patient's fears and concerns. If you get distracted or preoccupied while listening to a patient, become aware of that voice inside of you. Don't berate yourself. Recognize that you've gotten off track and then go back to listening wholeheartedly. "Here he goes again" is not an uncommon thought when we don't want to listen to someone; however, if we are hearing the same stories and complaints over and over again, it's probably because we never really listened the first time and the patient knows it. Really listening to the story for the hundredth time and suspending judgment for the hundredth time will go a long way to bridging the separateness between you and the patient.

Becoming a listener who can "be there" for someone is vital to achieving magic moments. It is a hard task yet the rewards are great for both patients and caregivers.

The Quakers refer to this as "devote listening"—giving someone our full attention without thoughts of judgment. It is not just listening with your ears; it is listening with your heart. Visualize the messages you receive coming straight into your heart.

Misunderstandings arise as a result of poor communication and listening skills. If you are in doubt about what someone is saying, it's important to clarify what is being said.

I once worked with a patient who I believed took up too much of my time. Usually she complained that she wanted someone in her room to help her.

On one occasion, she came out into the hallway and said, "Get to my room to help me now."

I had just been in her room and had ten other patients to get to, so I rushed by her and said, "I need to get to these other patients first. Please be patient."

I found out later that what she actually said was "Get her out of my room now."

Another patient in her room (who had a dementia) was destroying the room.

When we are under stress and pressure, we only hear what we want to hear. We don't take time to truly listen. If I had truly listened to this patient, I could have had a magic moment, prevented two patients from being upset and had less of a mess to clean up in the room. At the time, I believed the patient was interfering with my ability to focus on my tasks. I now believe that patients are our only task and their needs come first.

When to Talk or Listen

When is the best time to talk and listen to patients? Is it when we are in the hallway, at their bedside, taking them down to treatment or providing treatment in their room? The answer is all of the above. Every moment we are with a patient has the potential to create the type of magic that will bring meaning to our work.

It can happen when we least expect it, so we need to be open to creating more moments of listening and keeping the lines of communication open at all times.

Most people just want to be heard, have a chance to tell their story without judgment—a chance to be recognized for what and who they are. They need to feel like they are not alone and that we accept what they are saying or not saying. We deem "fixing" to be more valuable than listening, so our automatic response is to do or fix something. If we focus only on the fixing, however, we lose another opportunity to serve and heal with our gift of listening. We need to listen first before taking appropriate action.

Saint Bernard of Clair says, "You wish to see; listen. Hearing is the step towards vision."

Fifty-year-old Mr. Johns had a brain tumor and had surgery to remove it. The surgery went well, however, the surgical site did not close properly afterwards and, as a result, air infiltrated his brain, causing some mild brain damage and other physical defects. It was a heartrending situation that left him with limited mobility. He spent a good part of the day in his bed. He needed to talk about who he was before and after the surgery. He told his story over and over again, with much anger and with very colorful, threatening words, which caused staff to feel helpless, fearful and frustrated. The staff could empathize with him to a point, yet most found it extremely difficult to be with him and sit with him through his "outbursts," as they described it.

As helpers, there was no way they could "fix" or change his situation and, as a result, staff would avoid him and minimize contact with him. They would make quick entries and exits to and from his room and avoid spending any extra time with him because they felt so helpless, inadequate and overwhelmed.

Months went by and Mr. John's "angry outbursts" increased. The staff continued to avoid contact with him while increasing their requests for more sedative medication. When a new house-keeper was hired, however, things started to change. The nursing staff encouraged me to talk to this housekeeper and find out why Mr. Johns was so calm while she was on shift.

At first, the housekeeper was defensive. "I still clean the room, you know," she stated.

I acknowledged the great work she was doing and asked her to tell me more about Mr. Johns.

She smiled and said, "I listen to Mr. Johns. I put my broom against the wall and pull up a chair—only for a moment, though. I listen, I look in his eyes and I let him know I see him."

I asked the housekeeper why she had decided to do that and why she wasn't afraid.

"He was there," she replied. "I saw him, heard him and saw myself."

I had no more questions. For once, there was nothing more to be said.

The staff noticed a decrease in Mr. Johns' outbursts because of his relationship with the housekeeper.

How many times do fears, frustrations and judgments limit our ability to truly be there during someone's distress and discom-fort? How many times do we avoid the situation because we don't know what to do to make it better, or we believe there is no way to make it better? We may even overlook the support staff, who can play a pivotal role in establishing healing relationships with our patients. This includes housekeeping, maintenance, physical and recreational therapy, dietary, and many other support staff. In healthcare, we sometimes forget the value of working as a team with all disciplines. Frontline nursing staff members aren't the only ones who can make a difference. We need each other to serve others. When we are unable to make a connection with a patient, someone else on the team may be able to help.

Questions to Ponder

- Who are the people you identified as difficult to listen to? (Hopefully, you identified them in your listening exercise.)
- What makes them difficult for you to listen to?
- What thoughts cross your mind when you're attempting to listen to these people?
- When you hear yourself labeling patients as "complainers," "manipulators," "liars," "obstinate," "irritating," know-it-alls," or when you hear yourself saying, "I have heard this before," it means you no longer want to listen. Are you reacting to what patients have said, or just accepting what they said without inner commentary? Heartfelt listening occurs when we get out of our own way.

Jargon-Free Information

Clear communication is essential in building a rapport with our patients. We must not only "see" and "hear" them but acknowledge their concerns and consider what kind of comfort we can provide. We must also provide them with clear, sincere, concise, honest, jargon-free information like "We are here to help you. We will work on this together."

Sometimes, however, we use language that only we understand. We also tend to make assumptions that those in our care (or their family members) know what is going on and what to expect.

A family brought their loved one into the emergency room. They were unsure what was happening to him and only knew that he suddenly became unconscious. They were in distress and overwhelmed by fear that their loved one was dying. They believed he was receiving good care but wished someone would sit down with them and tell them what was going on.

People need and want information, especially when they feel they are not in control of a situation. In our efforts to help those in need, we may inadvertently forget that family members also need support and information. Even though they may not be directly involved in the patient's care, they are a valuable and integral part of the big picture and deserve to have all the information concerning their loved one.

Unfortunately, we often feel threatened or burdened by this kind of discussion. We are not always comfortable acknowledging (to ourselves or others) that we don't know all the answers. Are we okay with not having all the answers? Are we okay with letting those in our care know that we do not have the answers at this time? Can we reassure them that we will keep looking at ways to help and provide answers? We may feel that people are questioning our actions, judgments and competence. That little voice in our head says, "Aren't we doing enough? We are trying our best. They wouldn't understand." While this may well be the case, there are always ways to improve the situation and avoid further strain on ourselves and the family.

If we have trouble with this notion of helping and supporting the family with information and care, we should ask ourselves this question: if that was our loved one in the treatment room and we were in the waiting room, how would we like to be included?

Would it be out of line to ask for or impart information or seek support?

Questions to Ponder

- How do you decide who needs information?
- Who is your patient?
- How do you view a family's inquiry about the care of their loved one? Do you sometimes find yourself becoming defensive? Are you suspicious that the families are really looking for fault? Do you view their concerns with an open, understanding, compassionate attitude?

This same family's loved one was transferred to another hospital. While the family was sitting in the emergency room, a healthcare provider came out to introduce himself.

"My name is Bruce," he said, "and we are moving him to ICU." Bruce informed the family what tests they were performing and that they didn't know what was going on. He explained that when their loved one was stabilized, or if something changed, he would come and get them.

After receiving that one-minute explanation and acknowledgment, the family's perception about their situation immediately changed. Although their loved one later died, they remembered that they had been seen and heard. Unfortunately, they also remembered the less-than-compassionate care they had received at the previous hospital.

Using a person's name and introducing yourself are powerful communication tools. Knowing that someone has personally taken the time to introduce himself is comforting and respectful in an environment that often seems impersonal. Instead of rushing into a patient's room, why not take a few seconds to gently tap on the door and say your name? These few seconds are fundamental for creating magical helping encounters. As often as possible, stop and reflect on what and how you're doing something. If you do this, you will be honoring yourself and your patient.

I C YOU Method

I-Interest in the person is shown in the way you listen and respond
C-Concern-Let them know you are concerned and that you care
Y-"You"- Who you are as a person- the gift of your presence-your genuineness
O-Open, non-judgmental respectful attitude
U-Universal human need for compassion and kindness

The Importance of Body Language

A study from UCLA indicated that communication is more than just words. It is estimated that only 7% of any message is the spoken word, 38 % is voice quality (tone, tempo, intonation), and 55% is body language. This means that most of what we communicate is non-verbal.

As caregivers, we need to be aware of our non-verbal communication cues and those of our patients. Since we communicate 55% of the time without ever saying a word, we ought to be paying close attention to what our nonverbal signals are saying to patients. If you think you are too busy for a lesson in nonverbal communication, remember this: *you have the potential to irritate or soothe a situation with your very presence, every moment.*

Quite simply, whether you realize it or not, how you communicate with those in your care will determine the type of relationship you create with your patients. Do you respond impatiently with an annoyed voice? Do you hang out the door and into the hallway as you speak? Do you frequently look at your watch or become so preoccupied with your "tasks" of taking blood pressure and making beds that you leave a patient's room without any eye contact? In a conflict with an angry patient, do you automatically cross your arms over our body? Many times during my career as a nurse I forced myself to place my arms at my sides instead of across my chest. I knew that if I folded my arms across my chest when dealing with an aggressive patient I would only aggravate the situation. When I took a deep breath and hung my arms loosely at my sides (without clenching my fists!), I would begin to relax and so would my patient.

The SOOTHE Approach

Most of the people we serve suffer from some form of emotional or physical stress which affects their ability to receive our communication. If they are elderly, they may have hearing deficits. Some may be suffering from a mental illness that impairs their ability to cope and communicate.

The following tools will help you soothe almost any situation and lead you to more magic moments in your work:

S is for smile. A genuine smile helps relieve a patient's anxiety and aids in building trust. A smile can break down barriers and help build a foundation of warmth and caring.

O is for open-ended questions. Open ended questions are ones which cannot be answered with a yes or no. They help to provide understanding and clarity in a situation. Some examples: "What do you find most difficult right now?" "How can I best be of help to you right now?" Use the communication tool "reflection" to acknowledge the patient's emotional state and to help build trust. ("I can see this is bothering you.") Building trust is about doing what we say we're going to do. If we say we're going to come by their room, we must make sure we do so.

O is for open posture. This means no crossed legs, arms or hands. This conveys that we are approachable and willing to interact. Arms crossed over our chest can be intimidating or even condescending to patients.

T is for touch. A hand extended in greeting can provide comfort and reassurance. A hug or touch to the shoulder can convey compassion and understanding, especially when there are no words for the situation that we and the patient find ourselves in.

H is to halt your speech. Silence is an important tool that provides space for true heartfelt listening without judgment. Merlin in the movie *Excalibur* said, "You're not listening… well, your heart is not." Silence is a poignant form of communication. How comfortable are you with silence? Do you feel like you have to fill in every moment with talk?

E is for eye contact. Relating to another human being with our eyes conveys that we are interested, focused and concerned. By this I mean intermittent direct eye contact, not staring. We should be aware that in some cultures maintaining eye contact is a sign of disrespect. This was pointed out to me by a workshop participant who was of African descent. Avoid spending time focused on some task such as bed-making or jotting down information. Really look into the patient's eyes. Look at the person long enough to notice the color of his or her eyes. When sincere eye contact is made, time seems to stand still for both the patient and the helper.

Saying Goodbye

Even though it may be difficult, we should pay as much attention to the endings of our helping relationships as we do to building trust in the beginning. No matter how a relationship ends, there will likely be some degree of separation anxiety and grief. When a patient dies, goes home or is transferred, or when we are away for awhile, what can we say to the patient and family? What can we tell our patients that will be meaningful, respectful and will honor our professional relationship?

It is important to not rush through the ending of our helping relationships. Ending involves transition and change, and there is a natural and necessary psychological process that we go through. This process can involve excitement as well as grief, fear and anxiety. Often there are enormous fears in relation to dealing with the unknown or in leaving the known. Take a meaningful moment to explore with the patient some of his/her concerns and thoughts in regards to this transition. This will benefit both you and the patient. Explain what is going on and provide compassionate support. If appropriate and a referral for other help is indicated, ask yourself if there is anything you can do to ease the transition. If possible, introduce the patient to the other health professional who will be looking after him or her.

11

FINDING MEANING IN YOUR WORK

"Meaning is not what you start with, but what you end up with."

—PETER ELBOW

Finding meaning in our lives is a lifelong process of exploring the relationships we have with ourselves and others. Ann Belford Ulanov, author and Professor of Psychiatry at Christiane Brooks Johnson, said, "Meaning does not come to us in finished form, ready made; it must be found, created, received and constructed. We grow our way towards it."

So how do we, as healthcare providers, derive meaning from our work? This is a subject we don't often discuss or even acknowledge. Our meaning is closely tied to our values and our ability to be compassionate and kind. Unfortunately, healthcare workers may feel undervalued and underappreciated. Somewhere along the way, our work may have lost meaning and we no longer feel the satisfaction we initially felt in our career. As a result, we feel less compassionate. We complain that if we had more time and resources we could make meaningful contact with our patients and not be so rushed. We equate time with meaning, and miss the magic of those timeless moments when we connect with patients and know that we have made a difference in their lives. Our challenge then is to honor the meaning and essence of our work within the time (and budget) constraints of our present-day healthcare system. How can we do this? By focusing on what we *can* do each moment, and reframing how we perceive "time." When we focus on what we can't do, we miss the value in the most miniscule contact with our patients. When we perceive time as "lacking" or "in deficit," we bring more tension, agitation and anxiety upon ourselves. We need to appreciate and acknowledge every moment, create meaning in every moment. When a helper stops thinking ahead or fretting about the past and anchors him- or herself in the immediate presence of another human being in need, both the helper and the patient receive blessings that would have otherwise been missed.

Are you THRIVE-ing?

Before we can have a magical relationship with others, we must first have a magical relationship with ourselves. This means having encouraging and appreciative thoughts. So many times we are hard on ourselves: "I cannot answer one more call bell today or I will never get my report done and be able to go home. I must be a real poor time manager." "I am a complete failure and incompetent." It's crucial that we respect ourselves. In so doing, we also honor our work.

To help you honor every moment and *thrive* in your workplace, instead of just survive, ask yourself these questions:

T - Thoughts- How's your attitude?

Here - Are you present?

Relationships - Are yours respectful and kind?

Inspiration - Where/what is yours?

Values - Are yours guiding you?

Energy - Do you need to renew yourself?

Checking in to Thrive

Thoughts – Keep track of your thoughts during the day or for even one hour. Where does your mind tend to wander? Do you focus on the 10% that is not going right during the day? Part of your struggles with your thoughts has to do with your EGO. You spend so much of your day in reaction mode that you don't pause or believe you have no time to pause to see what you are reacting to. It can be one big chemically volatile situation. Your power lies in the ability to change first how you see the situation, then how you think and feel about the situation, and eventually how to take action (or not).

Here – Being there in the moments is easier said than done. The moments are not about time per se; it is about being present. What are you paying attention to? You aren't just putting in time. You are creating moments. Say to yourself: *I vow to give my full attention and presence to what I am doing or who I am with. I will not let myself be distracted by the past or the future in this moment.* Monitor your language? Are you living in the past or present? Beware of these key phrases: if only, could have, should have, would have, will be, must be, but, going to.

Relationships – Respectful relationships are essential in achieving satisfying work and a meaningful life. Are there times when you aren't very kind? Be honest with yourself. It may be hard to believe when you work in the helping field, but there are times when your kindness factor does become depleted. Building trust and listening are paramount to respect.

Inspirations – Inspire means "to breathe life into another." You need sources and places to go that take you beyond yourself and put you in touch with something bigger than yourself. This essentially is your spirit. This is where your relationship with your God, source, and creator can root and comfort you. Some people find this experience when they are out in nature. What grounds and anchors you in times of distress? What provides you comfort and hope? Can you create a place at work that has plants, trees, water and soothing music? Can you get out into the fresh air during the day? Cultivating creativity and intuition at work and in your life will be of benefit to you.

Values – This is where you identify what matters the most to you. Values are tied closely to your beliefs. Developing a personal mission statement begins by identifying what is important to you. Values can help guide you in making work meaningful or in identifying why you are doing what you are doing. Pitfalls can occur when what you say or do is incongruent with what you value. If you value patience and you find yourself behaving impatiently, you can become frustrated and anxious. Values are cornerstones of who you are and how you do things. They form the basis of how you see yourself and others, and how you interpret the world in general. Values can change through your experiences and it is important to revisit what you deem important.

Energy – Energy is fascinating and vital to a healthy and joyful life. Where do you go to renew yourself? Humor, play, and self care are some of the tools that help you boost your immune system, gain perspective, and ease and release tension. Is it possible for you to take your jobs seriously but yourself lightly? According to author Joel Goodman, "seven days without laughter makes one week." You need to refuel/refill all aspects of your whole self. Start by identifying the simple needs you have such as rest, relaxation, exercise and nutrition. Do you make sure you receive enough sleep? Are you skipping meals or breaks? It is a self-perpetuating cycle. You don't take time for yourself—a kind moment—and you may even berate yourself for not having a kind thought or action towards another. Can you find and create sacred kind moments for yourself at work?

When we are with a patient, why not be there in mind, body and spirit? Slowing down and bring a consciousness into all your tasks will bring meaning to your work. Even the most tedious tasks will have depth, texture and life if you honor every moment you're in the presence of a patient. In *Star Trek, Generations* movie, Malcolm McDowell says, "Time is a predator and we are its prey." Time seems to stand still when we are fully present and engaged, and when we are disengaged and distracted time seems to rush by. Make a note of how often in your shift time seems to rush by and how often time seems to stand still. Magic moments accentuate the preciousness of the timeless moment. Honor every moment, every snapshot in time, and refuse to be time's prey.

Questions to Ponder:

- How could we view time as a foe or a friend?
- What does it mean to experience "time of the heart"?
- Have you ever experienced moments where time seemed to stand still? When does this happen?
- How often you feel like your time's prey?
- When does time go "hunting" for you in your work?
- How do you know when you're time's prey? Do you experience more anxiety, irritability and feelings of inadequacy?

Your Values

"Your vision will become clear only when you look into your heart...Who looks outside dreams. Who looks inside awakens."

—Carl Gustav

When we operate our life in accordance with our deeply held personal beliefs—our values—we bring meaning into our lives. If we do not take time to reflect and focus on our values, we may feel uneasy and dissatisfied. When we function incongruently with our values, we become stressed. No amount of relaxation or meditation will ease these symptoms. We must realign ourselves with our truth, our values. Reacquainting ourselves with our values helps to create and honor Magic moments. Aligning ourselves with our values helps us to rediscover the meaning, the essence, of our work in healthcare.

Our values can and will shift throughout our lives, so it is critical to continually look at what we deem important. How can we identify what we value?

Imagine you have a big pickle jar and in that jar you place the following:

1) Five or six things in your work that are "big rocks"— things that you value and are really important to you.
2) The "gravel or sand" in your work—things that are not as important yet consume so much of your work that you can't fit the big rocks in
3) The "water" in your work—thoughts and/or actions that are drowning you

It's obvious that if you don't put in your "big rock" first, the gravel, sand and water will take over and there will be no room for anything else. Ironically, the "anything else" that gets left out are the words and moments in our work and life that are most important to us.

Exercise:

✓ Make a list of 20 values and then break them down into your top five vital "big rock" values. Below are some examples to get you started:

Abundance, achievement, accuracy, affluence, affection, acceptance, balance, benevolence, bravery, candor, calmness, certainty, cheerfulness, compassion, control, congruence, conformity, creativity, dependability, consistency, dignity, devotion, determination, effectiveness, expertise, excellence, exploration, enthusiasm, family, freedom, financial, flexibility, independence, generosity, health, honor, hygiene, humor, humility, investing, inspiration, leadership, learning, love, meticulous, order, optimism, outrageous, open-minded, professionalism, passion, peace, precision, punctuality, reliable, respect, recreation, reverence, resolution, reflection, relaxation, resilience, resourceful, restraint, service, smiles, skillfulness, silence, spontaneity, spirit, stability, success, thankfulness, trust, traditionalism, teamwork, uniqueness, usefulness, vision, victory, willingness, wonder, watchfulness, wisdom, zest.

Trudy had worked as a registered nurse for twenty-five years and complained of exhaustion and inadequacy.

Smiling weakly, she said, "I should have learned how to roller skate in my training. It would have saved time. I don't feel like I care as much as I used to. I don't feel like I have the time to care and I am too tired. I see a patient and all I think of is how much paperwork is tied up with this patient. For me, the paperwork is becoming more important than the patient."

She further explained that she used to be a kind, compassionate person however no longer was, as she was running on empty. Trudy identified kindness and compassion (in her relationships with her patients) as core values, and believed they had subsided. We explored how she could become more aligned with these values at work. She believed it wasn't possible, citing "This is just the nature of nursing and healthcare today."

I asked her what was different today from when she had first started her career. She said that then she had more time to be kind to the patients. She equated time with compassion and kindness. She believed she now had no control over her shift and that something "external; the administration" controlled her experiences every day. Trudy concentrated so much of her energy on the anticipated paperwork that she wished "It would just go away." She was focusing on the future and the past and was never in the present, where she could have had an amazing influence. She knew she wasn't being kind. She claimed that she never took time to chat with patients and avoided eye contact with them because "The look of need in their eyes was so overwhelming. Besides, I had other patients to attend to and didn't have the time."

I encouraged her to try an experiment of sorts, where she would consciously take a moment to acknowledge the patient and his/her concerns. She was not sure she could do this.

"Not enough time. We are short-staffed," she insisted.

After some hesitation, she agreed to anchor herself in the moment and focus directly on the present needs of the patient by looking at the person directly and acknowledging his/her fears and concerns.

When I saw her again a few weeks later, she said, "Centering myself with my breath helps me focus on the present, and, you know, my brief eye contact and smile seem to ease the agitated patients." She smiled and said, "I guess my compassion was always there. I just wasn't honoring it." She gave me a sly smile and added, "The paperwork is also there. We still don't have enough staff and I know it isn't going away, but this won't be the focus of my work. I believe I can be compassionate and efficient at the same time."

We discussed the definition of "efficient," which is being productive with minimum waste of effort and producing an effect. Peter Drucker, political economist and management guru, said that "efficiency is doing things right; effectiveness is doing the right things." In my view, we are being extremely efficient and effective when we are compassionate and can make a difference in another person's life.

Our words and thoughts are so powerful they create our reality. Our language and thoughts greatly influence how we cope with situations. We believe we are cognizant of how important thoughts and words are in our lives, yet we still use discouraging and paralyzing words. Using phrases such as "not possible" and "just the way it is" only complicates an already difficult situation.

Our attitude towards work also affects how we feel and act. If we regard work as a "necessary evil," we will be unfulfilled. If we consider work a blessing, we have the potential to be co-creators of Magic moments!

Questions to Ponder

- What are some of thoughts that may prevent you from being aligned with your values and creating meaning?
- What values and thoughts can you substitute for some of your defeating thoughts? For example, replace "I don't have enough time to make a difference," with "I have enough time to make a difference and I do this by... " Take an appreciative, positive approach instead of a deficit approach to your work.
- Where are you putting your time, energy and thoughts? Are they aligned with your beliefs and values?

Creating a Mission and Vision Statement

As healthcare workers, we must define what we want to bring to the people we serve. The best way to do this is to develop mission and vision statements. Our *mission* is defined as who we are now and the purpose we bring to our day-to-day work—how we want to make a difference. Our *vision* is where we want to go in our service as healthcare workers and how we will accomplish our mission. Both of them should be realistic.

During a critical incident stress debriefing with some emergency medical professionals, I asked what they thought their helping mission was. One young EMT immediately replied with authority and conviction, "No one was going to die on my shift."

I couldn't help to think that he was setting himself up for a career of hardship and additional stress with his difficult, unrealistic mission of helping. Because of the very nature of his work as an emergency medical professional, it was likely that people would die on his shift.

Our mission and vision statements must be attainable. We will only complicate our helping life if we set unrealistic expectations that are closely tied to how we derive meaning in our work. Examples of realistic mission statements are: "During my work I will treat everyone with an open, respectful, compassionate, patient attitude;" and "I will use my knowledge, skills and sensitivity to help my patients."

Mission statements will need to be revisited often —not just every year but several times a day. They remind us why we do this work, how we make a difference, and that we are, in fact, making a difference. Mission and vision statements serve as a compass. When we feel like our whole helping life is falling apart, they remind what we can and can't do. As Edward Everette Hale's wisely said, "I am only one, but still I am one. I cannot do everything, but still I can do something. And because I cannot do everything, I will do the something that I can do."

Questions to Ponder

- Think back on times in your work when you knew you were making a difference. How did you know? Was it with a patient you liked or someone you identified as being "difficult"?

- What made you make the extra effort? What was the extra effort?
- What does it feel like to reflect back and remember those moments?
- What is my work all about?
- What difference do I make?
- What can I influence?
- How do I bring value to my work?

Exercise:

- ✓ Take a moment to write down your personal helping mission and vision.
- ✓ Identify what you want to bring to your work and how you want to do that.

12

MINDFULNESS AND OPENNESS

"Where there is an open mind, there will always be a frontier."

—CHARLES F. KETTERING

Mindfulness

Mindfulness is essential on our journey of creating magic moments in healthcare. Practicing mindfulness helps to release us from the torments of our mind. We become more aware of the beauty of the immediate, the present situation we find ourselves in, for that is really all we have. Children are naturally inquisitive and pay attention to the miracles unfolding around them, however, adults seem to take things for granted. We have all had experiences where we suddenly notice something and wonder if it had always been there. It could be a sign on the road or the sun setting on a tree or a picture on the wall. It makes us wonder how much we have missed. This consciousness, this mindfulness, being aware, being awake and full of gratitude for all we see, hear and observe around us, will lead us to appreciating the essence of each moment and breath we take.

Because mindfulness is in direct contrast to our hurried approach, we must continually practice it to avoid going off track. In his book *Coming to your Senses*, Jon Kabot Zin indicated that mindfulness is pivotal in our life and work. It is a consciousness, a moment-to-moment nonjudgmental awareness that is relaxed, where we are more clear and aware of our choices. Mindfulness is a process of observing, describing and paying attention without judging or criticizing the present moment. It helps direct our attention to one thing only and offers opportunity for acceptance and wisdom.

When we go within and focus on bringing light and energy to different parts of our body, we are focusing in the moment. I affectionately call this "BS with an extra S"—Breathing, Smiling and Stillness. So, when someone says that magic moments are all BS, say, "Yes it is, but with an extra S!"

Dr. Carl Rogers' description of "unconditional positive regard" (discussed in Chapter six) underscores the importance of breathing in achieving mindfulness:

The most basic mindfulness practice is available to anyone at any time, any place; sitting comfortably and concentrating on breathing. As we breathe in and out, it is important to notice the thoughts and feelings crowding the mind. They affect daily life, whether or not we are conscious of them. With practice, we can learn to let the thoughts and feelings come and go the way we breathe in and out, without being judgmental of ourselves. For instance, if we are feeling guilty, helpless or angry we can acknowledge without judgment and release the emotions at the same time. In practical terms, this helps to clear the mind so we can make better choices when dealing with people and situations.

In medical terminology, a genuine smile is referred to as a "zygomatic" smile. (That word alone should bring a smile to your face!) Can we tell the difference between a genuine smile and a phony one? According to Dr. Martin Seligman, author of *Authentic Happiness*, there are two kinds of smiles: the "Duchenne smile" and the "Pan American" smile. Seligman describes the two smiles as follows: "The first, called the Duchenne smile (after its discoverer Guillaume Duchenne), is genuine. The corners of the mouth turn up and the skin around the corners of the eyes crinkles (the crow's feet). …The other smile, called the Pan American smile (after the flight attendants in television ads for the now-defunct airline), is inauthentic."

Never underestimate the importance of a smile. Smiling takes fewer facial muscles than frowning and creates a warmth, acceptance and lightness to our relationships with ourselves and others. When we smile, we feel a sense of release. When someone smiles at us, we feel grateful. When we are in quiet contemplation, it helps to open the lips and mind to a gentle smile.

Another tool that allows us to capture Magic moments and mindfulness is stillness. One of my favorite quotes on stillness comes from the Bible: "Be still and know that I am God." For me this serves as a poignant reminder to bring stillness into my life and work, and in doing so, I become more conscious and present. Stillness occurs when we quiet our minds and stop our busy thoughts. It is in these quiet moments that we are able to check in, reframe and renew the value in our work. In his wonderful poem, *Natural Great Peace*, poet Nyoshul Khen Rinpoche said, "This mind is like a glass of muddy water. Stir it up and it becomes cloudy. Let it settle, calm and it becomes clear." More benefits and strategies of stillness are discussed in the helper's self renewal section.

Questions to Ponder

- What ways can you practice mindfulness in healthcare?
- How does practicing mindfulness help us in our work?
- How can you bring more Breathing, Smiling, and Stillness (**BSS**) into your work?

Openness

When we are open, we fear less and live more. We are curious and available to the possibilities of learning and gaining wisdom. We suspend judgment and are sincerely interested in everything around us. According to Wayne Teasdale, a Catholic monk and author, "Openness is receptivity to everyone and everything. It is quite fundamentally an 'other-centeredness,' a disposition of availability to others."

Belleruth Naparstek, psychotherapist and author who focuses on guided imagery, says, "Heartful practice is about keeping the heart open to the world around us, to people, places, ourselves and the divine, It means coming from a place of empathetic attunement, it is about seeing the connections, the interlocking webs of energy and among people and things and residing as much as possible in that place of no separation."

When we label things or people, it interferes with the essence of what really is and our ability to be open to the possibility of healing and connecting with our patients.

Exercise

✓ Observe a chair or an object without saying what it is. Do you experience a sense of vastness, amazement, and wonder? (This is the openness and receptivity that allows our heart to connect.)

✓ Observe patients without saying their name, describing them, or labeling them by their illness. What did you experience? Most likely you experienced their pure essence, a true connection.

A colleague and I were both feeling very frustrated, overworked and overwhelmed. I was short on openness and questioned why I was doing this work. I complained that I had no time to respond to a patient who was ringing the bell.

My colleague looked up at me, smiled and said, "You would think we had nothing to do all day but help these people."

My colleague's statement served as a poignant reminder of why I am here—to serve people in my care and be open to those moments to do so, no matter how inconvenient I deem them to be.

Our openness is sometimes in direct contrast to our need to have certitude in our work. Many of our daily decisions depend on our accuracy and judgment. We feel pressure from ourselves and those in our care to have absolutes and guarantees. We forget that there is value in being open to choices, approaches and possible treatments.

Most people want and believe they need a 100% guarantee, but the truth is that we don't always have the answers. As you know, there are no absolutes in our work. We are called upon to make judgment calls every day. Rigid, controlling, black-and-white-type personalities are common in health care workers. These personality traits can be extremely helpful in crisis situations that require quick decisions. Unfortunately, however, these traits can cause us extra strain as well as keep us from being truthful with our patients.

Telling our patients that we don't know the answer is just being "authentic." If we ask questions, the answer will appear. Asking questions allows ideas, solutions, possibilities, and creative experiences to emerge and flourish. This is the antidote to certitude thinking and encourages us to be seekers. Being a seeker is more than just asking questions; it is about searching, observing and exploring. We won't always have the answers, but we can search out the answers together.

When we wonder and are open, we are able to gain wisdom and insight and provide better compassionate care. Jose Ortega Y Gasset, author and philosopher said, "To be surprised, to wonder, is to begin to understand." In healthcare we are not always encouraged to wonder and we think we're expected to know and maybe even pretend that we do. There is tremendous value in acknowledging that we do not know and then we allow ourselves to be open, to wonder and to search for understanding.

Questions to Ponder

- How comfortable are you with not knowing?
- How often do you see the patient as "the other" instead of "we" and "us?"
- How available are you to those you deem as difficult or different?
- Do you usually think you know how things will turn out? What do you need to be more of? What do you need to be less of?
- How can you encourage openness and wonder in your work?

13

NURTURING AND SELF - RENEWAL

"One has to find a balance between what people need from you and what you need for yourself"

—Y'ESSYE NORMAN

One day, during my wellness presentation for caregivers entitled "A Life Well Lived," I asked the participants what would happen if they stopped what they were doing once in a while. The participants were encouraged to take a break and rest from their pace and busy life and work. In the back of room a hand went up and a younger caregiver responded, "It would scare the hell out of me to stop. Then I would really have to look at my life." She went on to say, "I am busy looking after myself, though. I jog four miles a day and work out for an hour in the morning and volunteer for three different nonprofit organizations."

The notions of self-renewal and nurturing can be foreign concepts to healthcare professionals. We are usually the last ones to realize that we have to stop and look after ourselves. We may not even be aware that we are withering away. Everyone else may notice that we are falling down the slippery slope of exhaustion, but we continue on in our work and life, pretending that everything is okay. We caregivers are notorious for forging ahead at our own peril. We are "super doers." We burn ourselves out trying to live up to our patients' (and our own) high expectations. When we're ill, we admonish ourselves for being under the weather. We work long hours and push ourselves hard, mentally and physically, with limited resources, under technical, time and political pressures.

Recently, I had some health challenges and scares, all within a three-month timeframe. It started off with a breast core biopsy for a suspected malignancy. The doctors claimed they were just being careful, since my mother is a breast cancer survivor. Then I had surgery for squamous cell carcinoma on my lip for the second time. Shortly after this, I put my back out, and my sciatica was crippling. (This was from an injury I had experienced during the birth of my second son twelve years earlier, which had not really bothered me since.) Even walking was difficult. Shortly after that, I felt rundown and got strep throat. That was it. I had a meltdown.

Of course, cumulative stress had been the primary cause of my situation. Being honest with my thoughts, feeling and emotions and seeking support and ways to nurture myself went by the wayside as I attempted to "buck up."

None of what we have discussed in this book will matter if we don't encourage self-nurturing amongst all healthcare workers. Nurturing and self-care need to be one of our "big rock" values. We will have nothing to give others if we don't develop ways to practice reflection and self-nurturing.

In Anne Bromley's article, Dr. Matthew Goodman, who teaches mindfulness at the University of Virgina, states the following: "Patients need healthcare professionals to be well enough themselves to be in a healing space... If we're rushed, stressed and overworked, it's hard to connect with patients with compassion and empathy. We can retain our technical skills, but the compassion goes..."

The Quiet Voice Within

Self-care is about creating reservoirs for ourselves that we can tap into when we feel exhausted and depleted. If we don't take care of ourselves, we simply won't be able to function properly in our jobs.

What do we need to do to nurture ourselves? In addition to looking after our physical bodies, we need to pay attention to our mind, spirit and emotions. I believe our wellness comes from within. We need to take time to listen to our quiet voice inside, the voice we may hear but choose to ignore. We can only hear this quiet voice when we stop and reflect.

Prayer and meditation can bring us comfort and peace during times of stress. Prayer takes us beyond ourselves and connects us with our divine source, God, creator, etc. You may find Theologian Reinhold Niebuhr's famous serenity prayer helpful when coping with stressful situations:

God, give us the serenity to accept what cannot be changed;
Give us the courage to change what should be changed;
Give us the wisdom to distinguish one from the other.

Asking for Help

We helpers are notorious for not asking for or accepting help. Asking for or accepting help from others is difficult for most caregivers because it makes us feel vulnerable. We prefer to do the helping. That way, we feel like we're in control of the situation. Frustration sets in when we realize we cannot help everyone and that some people don't want to be helped. It gets even worse when (and if) we realize that we need more help than those we are assisting. This is a tough situation because it goes against everything we believe in. I always tell myself that there will come a time in my life when I will need to receive more than I will be able to give. I hope I will have the insight to allow myself to receive someone else's magnanimous support and spark. Thank goodness for all those fire-starters!

Albert Schweitzer, medical missionary and Nobel Peace Prize winner, said, "At times our own light goes out and is rekindled by a spark from another person. Each of us has cause to think with deep gratitude of those who have lighted the flame within us."

Each time we hesitate to ask someone for help, we should ask ourselves this question: Who will we be if we can only give and not receive? Of course, the answer is: We will be downtrodden, exhausted, negative, and physically or emotionally ill. There is enormous value in knowing when to ask for help. Ideally, we won't wait until we are so depleted that we can barely find the energy to ask for help. We have to find ways in our life to share our burdens and allow others to occasionally help us carry our load. It is beneficial to identify those people who can be of assistance and who can support and/or rejuvenate us when we need it.

This notion of giving and receiving may be confusing to you. You might not realize a crucial fact—that *every time* you give, you can also receive. How is this possible? The key to receiving is being open to the possibility while you are giving and then allowing yourself to experience it. Try it! Ask yourself the following question: "Is this helping encounter an opportunity to renew myself, or will it drain me further?" If it drains you, look more closely to see if you inadvertently missed an opportunity to receive.

Questions to Ponder

- How do you know when you need help?
- Do you allow yourself to receive help?
- Is it okay for you to say no to someone who needs something that you're not able to give?
- When you're no longer able to give, do you know where to go for help?
- Do you know when to pass the torch to someone else so you can replenish yourself and continue the work of helping others?
- Do you believe that you are the only one who can help others and work that extra shift to be there for someone, when you have already worked twelve hours?
- How can you receive when you give? What would you receive?

Self-Acknowledgement

Helpers don't usually have difficulty acknowledging others' strengths, successes, and triumphs. We find it easy to encourage others to forge on and acknowledge their accomplishments. We are very good at patting others on the back. What we find challenging is giving *ourselves* acknowledgment and compliments and celebrating our successes. It's easier for us to accept self-criticism. We can become very critical and judgmental about ourselves and others. We may confuse self-acknowledgement with conceit and arrogance. When we receive a compliment or congratulations, we often devalue it and say something like, "Oh, it is not that important. It is really nothing."

Acknowledging ourselves is an integral component of self-renewal and our greatest gift to others. Our challenge is seeing self-acknowledgment as a positive, life-affirming way to nurture ourselves so that we can nurture others.) Like everyone else, we can learn from our difficulties. We need to teach and encourage ourselves to pay attention to what we do well and learn from those experiences that I call our "stretches." .We need to acknowledge, compliment and be kind to ourselves (and others) every single day. Loretta La Roche, a professional speaker on stress management, calls this "TAH DAH-ing." She asks us to stop TO-DOing and start TAH DAHing! There are many things that we do well and accomplishments we can be proud of. Even in moments of pain and struggle there will be positive components that we can accentuate and acknowledge. For some this may be as simple as "I got out of bed this morning!"

As we adopt self-acknowledgment as an integral tool in self-care, let's allow the following message from author Marianne Williamson to resonate through us and bask in the knowledge that we are truly meant to shine:

"Our deepest fear is not that we are inadequate. Our deepest fear is that we are powerful beyond measure. It is our light, not our darkness, that most frightens us. We ask ourselves, who am I to be brilliant, gorgeous, talented, fabulous? Actually, who are you not to be? You are a child of God. Your playing small does not serve the world. There is nothing enlightening about shrinking so that other people won't feel insecure around you. We are all meant to shine, as children do. We were born to make manifest the glory of God that is within us. It is not just in some of us; it's in everyone. And, as we let our own light shine, we unconsciously give other people permission to do the same. As we are liberated from our own fear, our presence automatically liberates others."

Dr. Nansook Park and colleagues found that gratitude, optimism, zest, curiosity, and the ability to love and be loved are the characteristics that most closely relate to life satisfaction. Let's acknowledge some of our positive traits and identify ones we want to work on in order to have a more joyful life.

Exercise

- ✓ Make at list of what you do well. Remember and repeat the encouraging voices and compliments that do come your way.
- ✓ Keep compliments, letters, awards, accomplishments and notes in a special place where you can review and revisit.
- ✓ Identify what specific behaviors, attitudes and beliefs have led to your success in life.
- ✓ Write down what you are most proud of.

The Replenishing Ring

In order to maintain a balance in our lives, it's important to nurture ourselves in all aspects of our lives: physically, mentally, emotionally and spiritually. If we nurture only one or two aspects and neglect the others, we will suffer, so it is important to search out ways to rejuvenate all of them.

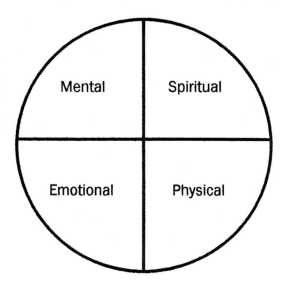

Physical—Our bodies speak to us in many ways, but we don't always pay attention. Helpers are notorious for working when they are "under the weather." Pay attention to your body and give it the rest, exercise and nutrition it needs.

Emotional—Acknowledge and accept a wide range of feelings in yourself and others. Find healthy ways to openly express and cope with your feelings. Look for ways to develop positive self-esteem.

Mental—This is our intellectual self—how we plan, write and think about things. This area is an opportunity to expand and grow from experiences and challenges. Read or take a course in something you find provocative, informative, enlightening, relaxing or challenging. Learn something new or relearn something that you have forgotten.

Spiritual—This is about getting in touch with something greater than you are and a willingness to seek meaning and purpose in human existence. For some of you, this might mean having a relationship with God or a higher power. For others, this could mean getting out in nature and exploring the world around you.

To me, wellness and renewal come from within. It is paying attention to that silent voice inside us and talking a quiet moment to check in with ourselves with awareness. It is about honoring all aspects of ourselves, especially the parts that may have been neglected. Wellness is a tremulous balance in response to continually changing internal and external demands of our world. I find I refuel myself when I am out in nature. I especially love being around my animals and riding my horse. Yoga has also become an integral part of my self-care as it fills all aspects of my replenishing ring. I take every opportunity I can to create stillness and silence, and to meditate, reflect and pray. I also believe showing gratitude to life and all its mystery is integral to my wellness.

Exercise

- ✓ Take a moment now to fill in your Replenishing Ring
- ✓ How do you presently deal with each of these areas of your life?
- ✓ Identify what you need to do to meet/replenish the needs of those areas.

The Four Rs (Recognize, Respond, Replenish, and Renew)

The Four Rs is a process that can help us institute renewal in our daily life.

- **Recognize**- Pay attention to those symptoms that tell us we are in need of refueling that lead to our exhaustion (see Chapter 4). Negativity, exhaustion and frequent physical illnesses are common signs.
- **Responding**- Now that we are paying attention and can identify our symptoms of exhaustion or need, we must honor ourselves and respond to *our* needs instead of those of others.
- **Replenishing**- We must refuel/refill all aspects of our *whole* self. Start by identifying the simple needs: rest, relaxation and wholesome food (We must ensure we have enough sleep and that we don't skip meals or breaks.)
- **Renew**- Once we have replenished, we must find ways to regularly renew ourselves so we can continue the work of caring for others.

Here are some ways to accomplish the Four Rs:

- **Take a 15-minute walk** during a lunch or coffee break. Take other opportunities to be physically active.
- **Eat sensibly.** Avoid excessive use of caffeine and alcohol. Drink plenty of water and juice.
- **Know and respect limits.** If you feel exhausted and need time off, it is important to take it. It is necessary to have regular time away from work.
- **Spend time with family and friends.** Talk to them. Listen to their concerns about your health and wellbeing.
- **Recreational and social activities** are important. Do things you love. Try something new.

- **Get some rest.** If insomnia is a problem, get up and do something relaxing or enjoyable.
- **Be on the lookout for any changes** in your habits, attitudes or moods. Don't ignore warning signals!
- **Share patients' and your reactions and issues** with colleagues. Don't hesitate to ask others for advice.
- **Include yourself on your list of people to care for.** Take time to do something for yourself every day. This will enhance your ability to give to others.
- **Make a gratitude list or keep a journal.** Keeping track of all there is to be grateful for can do wonders for your frame of mind.
- **Take time out**—Go out and explore the world around you! Think of it as an adventure in mystery, not mastery.
- **Enjoy music**- Music has tremendous healing benefits. Listening to soothing or inspirational music and learning how to play an instrument are wonderful ways to restore energy.
- **Make humor and play a priority.** Look for ways to bring more humor, play and "lightness" into your day.
- **Animals**- can nurture us with their unconditional acceptance and presence.
- **Take time for prayer and meditation**- These tools can provide comfort, inspiration and reassurance.
- **Be self-nurturing** and don't forget to laugh.

Magic Moment Mantras

Many, many thoughts go through our minds every day, the majority of which are usually negative and self-defeating. But there is a way to change this. By reading or repeating mantras— positive, life-affirming words and phrases—we can actually change the way we think about ourselves and our situation. (Mantra literally means "to free from the mind.")

There are two things to remember about mantras: the words or phrases you use must resonate with you; and they must be expressed in the present tense, as if what you are saying already exists. Here are some examples:

- I am patient
- I am open and accepting of my patients just as they are
- I am enough
- I have enough to make a difference
- I am peaceful
- I am compassionate
- I am finding humor
- I am taking myself lightly
- I make a difference
- I am accepting
- I am confident

In my own life I have found it helpful to consciously substitute self-deprecating and negative thoughts with something appreciative and positive. In my workshops, participants comment on how they are much more aware of their thoughts and how frequently their thoughts take on a self-deprecating tone. While writing this book I replaced negative thoughts like "I will never get this book done" and "There is nothing of value here" with "There is enormous value in this work" and "It is progressing perfectly."

Mantras help us counteract the thoughts, beliefs and assumption identified in the old baggage exercise. Consciously using mantras or affirmations helps to develop positive thoughts by using positive statements. We immediately start to feel more ener-

getic, inspired and encouraged. Experiment with the use of positive mantra yourself. See what happens!

14

CONCLUSION-WEAVING THE MAGIC

"Now this is not the end. It is not even the beginning of the end.
But perhaps it is the end of the beginning."

—SIR WINSTON CHURCHILL

Weaving is an ancient practice that has become the cornerstone for our culture throughout time. We are all weavers. Weaving is an apt metaphor for creation as it involves "bringing it all together." We may not recognize that we are weaving and may believe we are being woven by some external force over which we have no control. Every moment of every day we are weaving. As we weave our thoughts, various twists, turns and patterns of our life and work take shape. Some patterns repeat and some take us into new directions. I believe there is divinity in our weaving, whether we acknowledge it or not. The question is, what are we weaving into our life and work? Will it be our kindness, compas-

CONCLUSION-WEAVING THE MAGIC | 133

sion and presence? Will it be our listening ear? Will we weave in time to renew ourselves? For the past five years I have been weaving together ideas and stories for this book. There is no end to the tapestry of weaving this magic. I do not see the end. I see us adding our color, pieces and textures to healthcare as a whole. As you weave, you are creating a culture of caring. Yes, there are challenges and, with them come growth opportunities. When faced with hurdles, it is essential to weave through with awareness, consciousness and be gracious to yourselves and others. No two pieces of the tapestry are alike, and there is no one way to weave the magic.

It takes courage, practice, and tenacity to free yourself from debilitating thinking and responding. Looking at ways to bring out the best in you and in those you serve is not an easy task. Yet, it will probably be the most fulfilling and rewarding journey you will ever take. When you are feeling tired, lost, alone, and apathetic in your work, remember that you have the power to weave magic in ordinary moments. Take every opportunity to create magic moments, to serve someone in need using an open-minded and compassionate approach. These moments are like breathing—they happen even though we hardly notice they are happening. The sacred exchange of oxygen and the privileged exchange of serving another can be seen as mundane and ordinary or as "magic."

There is nothing more extraordinary than making a difference in someone else's life. Your every word and glance has the power to transform and ease another person's suffering. Each encounter with your patients, each exchange with your colleagues, can offer moments of awareness filled with grace, gratitude, growth and goodness. Never underestimate the power of your compassion, voice, smile and presence. They are the best tools you will ever have in healthcare.

In this book, I hope there was an opportunity for you to discover or rediscover, pause, reflect, renew, honor and remember your purpose as healthcare workers. I hope you feel just a little more inspired and insightful and now realize that you are the grand weaver of magic. I also hope this book serves as a new beginning for you and the incredible work that you do. May it be a catalyst in your continual exploration of finding meaning, purpose and inspiration in healthcare. I wish you many blessings on your journey as you create and honor the Magic around you!

 ☺

References

Adams, J. A., Murray R., (1998) The general approach to the difficult patient. *Emer Med Clin North Am,* 16: 689-700.

Covey, S. R. (1990). Seven *habits of highly effective People.* (1st. ed). New York: Simon & Schuster.

Bromley, A.. Mindfulness courses reduce stress amongst Doctors and Nurses-lead to more compassionate patient care. (2005) Retrieved September 2008 http://www.virginia.edu/insideuva/2005/02/mindfulness.html

Goldman, D. (2000). *Working with emotional intelligence.* United States: Bantam.

Ladner, L. (2004). *The lost art of compassion.* San Francisco: HarperCollins Publishers Inc.

Larson, D.G. (1993). *The helper's journey.* Champaign, Illinois: Research Press.

Muller, W. (1997) *How should I live.* United States: Bantam.

Remen, R. In service of life (1996) Retrieved October 2008 http://www.rachelremen.com/service.html

Schueman, H., & Thetford, W. (1976) *A course in miracle.* United States: The Foundation for Inner peace.

Sladden , J.. Does the whole in health care need to filled holistically BMJ Careers (2006) Retrieved October 2008 http://careers. bmj.com/careers/advice/view-article.html?id=1592

Stuart, G., & Sundeen S. J. (1979). *Principles and practice of psychiatric nursing.* St. Louis: The C. V. Mosby Company.

Tolle, E. (1997). *The power of now.* Vancouver British Colombia: Namaste Publishing Inc.

Zinn-Kabat, J. (2005) *Coming to our senses.* New York: Hyperion.

Zur, O. and Nordmarken, N.. To Touch Or Not To Touch: Exploring the Myth of Prohibition On Touch In Psychotherapy And Counseling (2008). Retrieved October 2008 http://www.zurinstitute.com/touchintherapy.html

Suggested Reading

Brady, M. (2003) *The wisdom of listening*. Boston: Wisdom Publications.

Dossey, L. (2006) *The extra-ordinary healing power of ordinary things*. New York: Three Rivers Press.

Dossey, L. (2000) *Reinventing medicine: beyond mind–body to a new era*. New York: HarperOne.

Dossey, B., & Keegan, L. (2008) *Holistic nursing: a handbook for practice (5*[th]*. Ed.)* Boston: Jones and Bartlett Publishers.

Frampton, S,. Gilpin, L., & Charmel, P. (2003) *Putting patients first: designing and practicing patient-centered care.* San Francisco: Jossey-Bass.

Ferrucci, P. (2006) *The power of kindness*. New York: Penguin Group.

Hanh, Thich Nhat. (1992) *Peace is every step*. New York: Bantam Books

Needleman, J. (1997) *Time and soul*. (1st. ed.) New Your: Doubleday Business.

Nichols, M. P. (1995). *The lost art of listening*. New York: The Guilford Press.

Pink, D. (2006) *A whole new mind*. New York. Penguin Group.

Remen, R. (1997) *Kitchen table wisdom: stories that heal.* New York: Riverhead Trade.

Rinpoche, C. N., & Shlim, D. R. (2004). *Medicine & compassion.* Somerville MA: Wisdom Publications Inc.

Zander,. R., & Zander, B. (2000) *The art of possibility.* United States: Harvard Business School Press

Magic Moments in Health Care-
Workshop Participant Reviews~

"Profound and dynamic workshop! I looked forward to coming to each session and felt energized after. I learned a lot about myself and others and I just love that. I now have an ability to go back and see a patient and myself in a new way."

"I think everyone in heathcare should take this course. I came in looking for new ways to be able to help patients I work with. I came out having a new purpose of what I do. Donna you do a great job looking at the whole picture and enlightening us. I can now evaluate myself."

"Excellent- encouraged self realization and gave me new ways to deal with certain patient situations."

"Great, very enjoyable and fulfilling, I am now able to see the patients with a more open nonjudgmental mind. You learned something new each session."

"I didn't think there was anything new I could learn. Wrong Wrong Wrong. I now know that you create "magic moments" by being more aware of others and accepting of others for who they are... and go on from there. "

"Awesome and inspiring helped me to take myself and my work to another level and I will continue to."

"Everyone could benefit for this course- amazing and enlightening. This was an opportunity for self reflections, and encouragement that we can make a difference. I now acknowledge that little thinks can make a difference. I am also now aware of how my own perceptions and attitudes color everything in my life and work."

"This is a precious workshop that encourages us to be better individuals and support our patients."

"A very important workshop for everyone. To stop and evaluate our connection with others."

"This course was an opportunity to do some team building and reflecting. Let do more of these workshops!"

"Donna I liked your approach. You are a person who has walked the walk."

"Exercises and group activities were very valuable. Donna's course did an excellent job of enabling us to think outside the box."

"I learned that I count and what I do is important and it helped me do my job better."

About the Author

Donna Devlin's passion is people and the human spirit. She is a contributing author of a book entitled "Awakening the Work Place Volume 2". Donna has a Bachelors degree in General Studies with emphasis on sociology and communications from the University of Calgary and is a Registered Psychiatric Nurse with twenty-five years of community experience. Donna has worked as therapist, consultant and educator for the Edmonton and Calgary Mental Health consulting teams and was responsible for developing and implementing an outreach response program for the survivors of the July 1987 Edmonton Tornado. Since 1997, she has operated a consulting service, offering keynote addresses, workshops, seminars and facilitation to nonprofit organization, private corporations, volunteer organizations, educational institutions, healthcare facilities and police services. She works as a grief consultant and educator for McInnis and Holloway, one of Canada's largest independent funeral homes. Donna has been interviewed on national television radio and newspapers. She is a speaker on the Calgary roster for LifeSpeak Inc, which is a national company dedicated to bringing valuable work-life balance workshops and streaming video clips to busy employees to help them thrive in all that they do.

In addition, Donna has been nominated for an international "Human Interaction Best Practice—Spirit of Caring" Award Donna is known as a gifted speaker who creates excellent learning environments with her open, engaging style, compassion and humor. She lives in the Alberta Rocky Mountains foothills with her husband, three children, two dogs, five horses, two cats and one fish.

If you would like to invite Donna to your workplace, staff retreat day, next conference or learn more about her and her workshops, please feel visit her website at www.donnadevlin.com.

Donna invites you to share your Magic Moment stories in health care by sending them to her via email to donna@donnadevlin.com.

ISBN 142517006-4

9 781425 170066